MEDICAL MALPRACTICE

MEDICAL MALPRACTICE

A PHYSICIAN'S SOURCEBOOK

Edited by

RICHARD E. ANDERSON, MD, FACP

Chairman and Chief Executive Officer,
The Doctors Company, Napa, CA

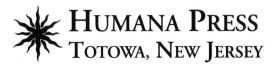

HUMANA PRESS
TOTOWA, NEW JERSEY

© 2005 Humana Press Inc.
999 Riverview Drive, Suite 208
Totowa, New Jersey 07512

humanapress.com

For additional copies, pricing for bulk purchases, and/or information about other Humana titles, contact Humana at the above address or at any of the following numbers: Tel.: 973-256-1699; Fax: 973-256-8341, E-mail: humana@humanapr.com; or visit our Website: www.humanapress.com

This book is sold with the understanding that neither the author nor the publisher is engaged in rendering legal advice or the practice of law. If legal advice is required, it is the responsibility of the reader to hire an attorney. Publisher and author are not responsible for any errors or omissions or for any consequences from the application of the information presented in this book pertaining to matters of law.

Due diligence has been taken by the publishers, editors, and authors of this book to assure the accuracy of the information published and to describe generally accepted practices. The contributors herein have carefully checked to ensure that the drug selections and dosages set forth in this text are accurate and in accord with the standards accepted at the time of publication. Notwithstanding, as new research, changes in government regulations, and knowledge from clinical experience relating to drug therapy and drug reactions constantly occurs, the reader is advised to check the product information provided by the manufacturer of each drug for any change in dosages or for additional warnings and contraindications. This is of utmost importance when the recommended drug herein is a new or infrequently used drug. It is the responsibility of the treating physician to determine dosages and treatment strategies for individual patients. Further it is the responsibility of the health care provider to ascertain the Food and Drug Administration status of each drug or device used in their clinical practice. The publisher, editors, and authors are not responsible for errors or omissions or for any consequences from the application of the information presented in this book and make no warranty, express or implied, with respect to the contents in this publication.

Production Editor: Robin B. Weisberg
Cover design by Patricia F. Cleary

This publication is printed on acid-free paper. ∞
ANSI Z39.48-1984 (American National Standards Institute) Permanence of Paper for Printed Library Materials.

Photocopy Authorization Policy:

Printed in the United States of America. 10 9 8 7 6 5 4 3 2 1

eISBN 1-59259-845-5

Library of Congress Cataloging-in-Publication Data

Medical malpractice : a physician's sourcebook / edited by Richard E. Anderson.
   p. ; cm.
  Includes bibliographical references and index.
  ISBN 1-58829-389-0 (alk. paper)
  1. Physicians--Malpractice--United States.
  [DNLM: 1. Malpractice--United States. 2. Insurance, Liability--United States. 3. Medicine--United States. 4. Physicians--United States. W 44 AA1 M4884 2005] I. Anderson, Richard E.
  KF2905.3.M439 2005
  344.7304'11--dc22

                                        2004008594

DEDICATION

This book is dedicated to the men and women in the medical profession who, day and night, care for the sick and comfort the dying.

PREFACE

Books such as this one are deceptively difficult to create. The general subject is neither happy, nor easy, nor most anyone's idea of fun. Malpractice litigation, however, has become a central fact of existence in the practice of medicine today. This tsunami of lawsuits has led to a high volume of irreconcilable rhetoric and ultimately threatens the stability of the entire health care system. Our goal has been to provide a source of reliable information on a subject of importance to all who provide medical care in the United States.

The book is divided into four sections. Part I gives an overview of insurance in general and discusses the organization of professional liability insurance companies in particular. Part II focuses on the litigation process itself with views from the defense and plaintiff bar, and the physician as both expert and defendant. Part III looks at malpractice litigation from the viewpoint of the practicing physician. Some of the chapters are broadly relevant to all doctors—the rise of e-medicine, and the importance of effective communication, for example. The other chapters are constructed around individual medical specialties, but discuss issues that are of potential interest to all.

Part IV looks ahead. "The Case for Legal Reform" presents changes in medical-legal jurisprudence that can be of immediate benefit. The final two chapters take a broader perspective on aspects of our entire health care system and its interface with law and public policy.

This book would not have been possible without the encouragement of Dr. Frank E. Johnson, and the collaboration of Drs. David B. Troxel and Mark Gorney.

I am indebted to each of the contributors for their effort, wisdom, and experience.

I owe special gratitude to Susan Baker for reviewing, editing, and coordinating the many pieces of the manuscript.

Richard E. Anderson, MD, FACP

INTRODUCTION

Richard E. Anderson, MD, FACP

It is a difficult time to be a physician in the United States. In an era when life expectancy is increasing, when major progress has been recognized in the prevention and treatment of coronary artery and cerebrovascular disease, when a new generation of biologic therapies is beginning to reward decades of effort in the battle against cancer, when AIDS has become treatable and preventive vaccines are entering clinical trials, when CAT scanning and MRIs have revolutionized our windows into the human body, when surgeons can utilize noninvasive operative techniques and robotic surgery is a reality, when science is now unveiling the genomic abnormalities in a host of human diseases, how can this be?

Although our therapeutic armamentarium has never been greater, the pressures on the practice of medicine seem to have increased even more. Physicians talk about "the coming medical apocalypse" *(1)*, ask whether we are "helpless" *(2)*, or whether "...being a doctor is still fun" *(3)*? Scholarly research is undertaken to measure the degree of physician discontent and dissatisfaction with the practice of medicine *(3–8)*.

Part of the problem lies in the tangle of conflicting messages physicians regularly hear. Although societal measures of health are improving, the incidence of medical error is said to be unacceptably high *(9,10)*. Malpractice litigation is said to target "bad" physicians and to be a necessary adjunct to regulatory and professional discipline *(11)*, yet nearly one in five doctors reports a malpractice claim annually and one-third to one-half of high-risk specialists face a claim every year. Are they all bad doctors? Plaintiff attorneys say they carefully screen malpractice claims before filing, yet 70–80% of these claims are still found to be without merit *(12)*.

In this book, we look in detail at contemporary medical malpractice litigation. We review its history, examine medical malpractice insurance (which has become a virtual necessity to protect physicians and indemnify injured patients), discuss specialty-specific issues, and, finally, explore alternatives to the current system.

MEDICAL PRACTICE IN THE NEW MILLENNIUM

Before focusing on these important concerns, let us look into the context of medical practice at the onset of the new millennium. Washburn *(1)* identifies five trends that he argues have brought us to the brink of a "medical meltdown":

1. Excessive business and legal complexity in the provision of medical care.
2. Decreased medical spending without reduced demand for medical services.
3. The increasing role of for-profit corporations in changing the traditional emphasis on patient care into concern for shareholder equity.
4. A growing population of uninsured patients adding to the financial stresses on physicians and health care institutions.
5. Provider demoralization.

Keeping pace with ever-expanding medical knowledge is a daunting task, but physicians must practice "under significantly expanded legal obligations, face stricter standards of professional accountability for medical negligence, and no longer enjoy exemption from the laws of competition" *(13)*. Doctors now face criminal penalties for, among other things, inadequate documentation, elder care deemed unacceptable, or erroneous emergency room triage *(1)*.

Concern over the rising cost of health care has led to the era of "managed care." It is difficult to find any constituency that is fully satisfied with this development. Physicians are alternately depressed and enraged at the erosion of their authority in offering professional judgments on behalf of their patients. Doctors across the United States applauded the American Medical Association effort to impose the same malpractice jeopardy on managed care organizations that they themselves faced. This "the enemy of my enemy is my friend" philosophy ultimately foundered with the realization that more litigation was a poor prescription for America's health care system. Physicians came to understand that these lawsuits would not exempt them from their own legal battles, but would instead add another cause of action to the malpractice allegations they already faced.

Government has made life more difficult for America's doctors with laws that have reduced Medicare spending by hundreds of billions of dollars without taking action to reduce demand for services. The federal government pays for approximately 45% of all health care in the United States *(14)*. Therefore, these actions have significant direct impact, and, in addition, reset the bar for the rest of the health care marketplace.

The rise of for-profit corporate medicine offered promise of numerous important advantages:

1. Funds for infrastructure investment, including the information technology in which health care lags far behind other industries.
2. The potential to offer more consistent outcomes and systematic quality assurance.
3. Scale to allow development of appropriate institutional and provider specialization.
4. Institutional personnel who could free physicians from activities not directly related to patient care.
5. The rationalization of a fragmented industry that would produce enhanced quality at lower cost.

Instead, most cost savings have come from simply reducing payments to providers. Quality has proven difficult to define and even harder to measure. Profit imperatives have led to greater selectivity in choosing which patients to service, rather than commitment to better processes for improved outcomes. Physicians have found it difficult to align their incentives with those of their employers, and employers have found it equally difficult to manage doctors.

Patients, nominally the designated beneficiaries of these changes, seem the unhappiest of all. They have lost the unquestioned assurance that the physician is their advocate. Shifts in the marketplace may force them to find new doctors without warning or cause. Medical costs are again rising rapidly, and patients are being asked to pay an increasing share of their own medical bills (15). Only 44% of Americans express "a great deal of confidence" in medicine (16). (It is of interest, although not reassuring, that only 12% have a similar degree of confidence in those who run law firms, and 15% in Congress).

More than 45 million Americans do not have health insurance, but physicians must provide care to all under legally and ethically defined circumstances. For the remainder of the population, a panoply of public and private health plans, not to mention laws and guidelines, regulate the provision of health care.

THE INCREASING IMPACT OF LAW AND REGULATION ON MEDICAL PRACTICE

The legal context of medical practice has changed significantly in recent years. The position of physicians within the US legal system is "neither as lofty nor as protected as it was previously" (13). There are new legal obligations, stricter liability laws, and increased competition. "Physicians are expected not to discriminate on the basis of race, national origin, or disability in the selection of patients or the provision of medical care; to participate in emergency care when part of corporate hospital enterprises; to conform their practices to a nationally based professional standard of care; to price their services competitively; and to not use illegal tactics to eliminate the competition" *(13)*.

The definition of standard of care has evolved from the practices of competent physicians in the community (the locality rule) to national standards as articulated in the medical literature and practiced anywhere in the country.

Contemporary concepts of informed consent are only 30 years old and are now based on fundamental principles of patient autonomy rather than physician judgment. Although health care as a right or a privilege may still be debated, our laws have increasingly defined the terms of access and the parameters of care.

Increasingly, legal standards of care of have replaced medical standards. In some cases this may be relatively explicit, such as indications for Cesarean section based more on the probability of liability than medical judgment. Frequently, however, the replacement of medical judgment by courtroom standards is more subtle. Examples are as varied as the high rate of "false-positive" readings on mammography and the high incidence of antibiotic prescription to prevent even the remotest possibility of Lyme disease *(17)*.

In either case, the outcome is similar, an increase in the practice of defensive medicine. This is unfortunate for two reasons. First, it adds to the cost of care and thereby reduces access *(18)*. Second, defensive medicine, by definition, is unnecessary. It undermines both the doctor–patient relationship and physician belief in the value of medical judgment.

THE PROFESSION OF MEDICINE

Therefore, it is not surprising that physician "angst" is high. Washburn says it plainly enough: "Ask any clinician: it is getting harder and harder to enjoy practicing medicine" *(1)*. More than one-third of doctors say they would probably not choose to enter medical school again *(3)*. Although 84% of women physicians express satisfaction with their career, 31% say they might not choose to be a physician again *(7)*. This is especially notable because of the rising percentage of America's doctors who are women. By 2010, the figure is projected to be 30% *(7)*.

The primary cause for this dissatisfaction is not declining income, but decreased autonomy and the sense that medical practice is no longer the calling it once was *(2,3,5,7)*. There is a major groundswell of comment on the nature of physician-hood, and the meaning of "profession" *(19–22)*. This admirable discourse illustrates the nature of the pressures impacting the practice of medicine. In the face of "perverse financial incentives, fierce market competition, and the erosion of patients' trust" *(19)* physicians are asked to re-emphasize their commitment to the profession of medicine. The three core elements of professionalism are defined as follow *(19)*:

1. Moral commitment to the ethic of medical service.
2. Public profession of values.
3. The negotiation of "social priorities that balance medical values with other social values."

This process will result in a new social contract between physicians and society.

The authors of the proposed Charter on Medical Professionalism *(23)* also see professionalism as the core of the social contract for medicine and are concerned that the pressures of contemporary medical practice are "tempting physicians to abandon their commitment to the primacy of patient welfare." They identify the following three fundamental principles:

1. Principle of primacy of patient welfare.
2. Principle of patient autonomy.
3. Principle of social justice.

The latter requires physician advocacy beyond the welfare of individual patients to "promote justice in the health care system" *(23)*.

Ten professional responsibilities are also cited:

1. Commitment to professional competence.
2. Commitment to honesty with patients, emphasizing both informed consent, and prompt reporting and analysis of medical error.
3. Commitment to patient confidentiality.
4. Commitment to maintaining appropriate relations with patients such as the avoidance of patient exploitation for sexual advantage, financial gain, or other private purpose.
5. Commitment to improving quality of care.
6. Commitment to improving access to care.
7. Commitment to just distribution of finite resources.
8. Commitment to scientific knowledge.
9. Commitment to maintain trust by managing conflicts of interest.
10. Commitment to professional responsibilities emphasizing the individual and collective obligations to participate in processes to improve patient care *(23)*.

In today's medical-legal world, there are no guarantees against unwarranted litigation, and no certain protection against continuing erosion of the doctor–patient relationship. Nonetheless, every constituency in our society agrees on the critical nature of medical services and all want more, not less, access. Ultimately, the practice of medicine is too important, and the men and women who undertake it too estimable, for the system not to balance itself.

This book is offered as a look at the problems, some solutions that are available today, and more that are possible in the future.

REFERENCES

1. Washburn ER. The coming medical apocalypse. The Physician Executive, 1999:34–38.
2. Davidson C. Are we physicians helpless. N Engl J Med 1984; 310:1116–1118.
3. Chuck J, Nesbitt T, Kwan J, Kam S. Is being a doctor still fun? West J Med 1993; 159:665–669.
4. Murray A, Montgomery J, Chang H, Rogers W, Inui T, Safran D. Doctor discontent—a comparison of physician satisfaction in different delivery system settings, 1986 and 1997. J Gen Intern Med 2001; 16:451–459.
5. Landon B, Reschovsky J, Blumenthal D. Changes in career satisfaction among primary care and specialist physicians, 1997–2001. JAMA 2003; 289:442–449.
6. Sullivan P, Buske L. Results from CMA's huge 1998 physician survey point to a dispirited profession. CMAJ 1998; 159:525–528.
7. Frank E, McMurray J, Linzer M, Elon L. Career satisfaction of US women physicians. Arch Intern Med 1999; 159:1417–1426.
8. Schulz R, Scheckler W, Moberg D, Johnson P. Changing nature of physician satisfaction with health maintenance organization and fee-for-service practices. J Fam Practice 1997; 45:321–330.
9. Kohn LT, Corrigan JM, Donaldson MS. To Err Is Human: Building a Safer Health Care System. Washington, DC: Institute of Medicine, 1999.
10. Weiler PC, Hiatt HH, Newhouse JP, Johnson WG, Brennan TA, Leape LL. A Measure of Malpractice. Cambridge, MA: Harvard University Press, 1993.
11. Nace BJ, Stewart LS. Straight talk on medical malpractice. American Trial Lawyers Association, 1994:20.
12. Harming Patient Access to Care: Implications of Excessive Litigation. Subcommittee on Health, Committee on Energy and Commerce, US House of Representatives. Washington, DC: U.S. Government Printing Office, 2002:160.
13. Rosenbaum S. The impact of United States law on medicine as a profession. JAMA 2003; 289:1546–1556.
14. Levit K, Smith C, Cowan C, Sensenig A, Catlin A, Team HA. Health spending rebound continues in 2002. Health Affairs 2004; 23:147–159.
15. Herper M. GE Strike Sounds Health Care Alarm. Forbes.com. Vol. http://www.forbes.com/home/2003/01/14/cx_mh_0114ge.html, 2003.
16. Taylor H. The Harris Poll #6, Confidence in leadership of nation's institutions remains relatively high: www.harrisinteractive.com/harris_poll/index.asp?PID=3, 2000.

17. Anderson R. Billions for defense: the pervasive nature of defensive medicine. Arch Intern Med 1999; 159:2399–2402.
18. U.S. Department of Health and Human Services. Confronting the New Health Care Crisis: Improving Health Care Quality and Lowering Costs by Fixing Our Medical Liability System. Washington, DC, 2002:1–28.
19. Wynia M, Latham S, Kao A, Berg J, Emanuel L. Medical professionalism in society. N Engl J Med 1999; 341:1612–1616.
20. Brennan T. Physicians' professional responsibility to improve the quality of care. Acad Med 2002; 77:973–980.
21. Swick H. Toward a normative definition of medical professionalism. Acad Med 2000; 75:612–616.
22. Meakins J. Medical professionalism in the new millenium. J Am Coll Surg 2003:113–114.
23. Brennan T, Blank L, Cohen J, et al. Medical professionalism in the new millennium: a physician charter. Ann Int Med 2002; 136:243–246.

CONTENTS

CONTRIBUTORS

RICHARD E. ANDERSON, MD, FACP • *Chairman and Chief Executive Officer, The Doctors Company, Napa, CA; former Chief of Medicine, Scripps Memorial Hospital, LaJolla CA, and former Clinical Professor of Medicine, University of California, San Diego, CA*

TROYEN A. BRENNAN, MD, JD, MPH • *Department of Health Policy and Management, Harvard School of Public Health, Brigham and Women's Hospital, Boston, MA*

MICHAEL JAY BRESLER, MD, FACEP • *Clinical Professor, Division of Emergency Medicine, Stanford University School of Medicine, Stanford, CA; Medical Director, Department of Emergency Medicine, Mills-Peninsula Health System, Burlingame, CA*

JONATHAN I. EPSTEIN, MD • *Professor, Departments of Pathology, Urology, and Oncology; the Reinhard Professor of Urologic Pathology; and Director of Surgical Pathology, Johns Hopkins Medical Institutions, Baltimore, MD*

EDWARD FOTSCH, MD • *Medem Inc., San Francisco, CA*

MARK GORNEY, MD • *Founding Member, Board of Governors, and Medical Director, The Doctors Company, Napa, CA; Professor (em), Plastic and Reconstructive Surgery, Stanford University, Stanford, CA*

FRED J. HIESTAND, JD • *Counselor at Law; General Counsel to the Civil Justice Association of California (1978–Present); CEO and General Counsel to Californians Allied for Patient Protection, Sacramento, CA*

DAVID WM. HORAN, MD, JD • *Trial lawyer, St. Louis, MO and Chicago, IL; Member of Trial Team, Miles vs. Philip Morris, US*

ANN S. LOFSKY, MD • *Anesthesiologist, Saint John's Hospital, Santa Monica, CA; Member, Board of Governors, The Doctors Company, Napa, CA*

JOEL A. MATTISON, MD, FACS • *Department of Utilization Management and Quality Assurance, St. Joseph's Hospital, Tampa, FL; former Clinical Professor of Surgery, University of South Florida, Tampa, FL*

MICHELLE M. MELLO, JD, PhD, MPhil • *Assistant Professor of Health Policy and Law, Department of Health Policy and Management, Harvard School of Public Health, Boston, MA*

WILLIAM M. SAGE, MD, JD • *Professor of Law, Columbia Law School, New York, NY*

JACK M. SCHNEIDER, MD • *Chief Medical Officer, Sharp Mary Birch Hospital for Women, San Diego, CA*

DAVID M. STUDDERT, LLB, ScD, MPH • *Department of Health Policy and Management, Harvard School of Public Health, Boston, MA*

DAVID B. TROXEL, MD, FCAP • *Member, Board of Governors, The Doctors Company, Napa, CA; Clinical Professor, Health and Medical Sciences, University of California, Berkeley, CA*

MALCOLM H.WEISS, MD • *Clinical Professor, Department of Family and Community Medicine, University of Nevada School of Medicine, Reno, NV*

I INSURANCE

1 Insuring the Practice of Medicine

Mark Gorney, MD
and Richard E. Anderson, MD, FACP

SUMMARY

Although all physicians are aware that practicing medicine in the United States is virtually impossible without some form of liability insurance, many have only a limited understanding of how the American system of professional assurance really works. It is important for the practicing physician to understand not only some of the technical language regarding insurance but also the various forms in which it is available. Doctors should understand the distinguishing features of an effective insurance program.

Key Words: Spread of risk; underwriting; claims made; occurrence; surplus.

INTRODUCTION

Virtually all practicing physicians in the United States require medical malpractice insurance. Although malpractice insurance is legally required in only a few states, the vast majority of hospitals and other health care institutions mandate that all medical staff members be insured. Specialty insurance companies that provide only professional liability insurance and multiline companies that cover this type of risk and many others provide this coverage.

From: *Medical Malpractice: A Physician's Sourcebook*
Edited by: R. E. Anderson © Humana Press Inc., Totowa, NJ

About two-thirds of America's doctors are insured by mutual or reciprocal companies. These are owned by the physician policyholders and are not responsible to outside shareholders. Virtually all of these companies specialize in professional liability insurance with limited or no exposure to other lines of business. The remaining one-third of doctors are insured by publicly traded commercial carriers owned by shareholders rather than policyholders. Most, but not all, of these companies sell multiple lines of insurance and tend to move in and out of malpractice coverage as business conditions warrant.

The fundamental business principles that apply to all American businesses also apply to insurance companies: income must cover expenses. For insurance companies, the major categories of expenses are as follows:

1. *Losses* represent the payments made to plaintiffs as a result of jury verdicts or settlements.
2. *Legal defense* represents the legal costs associated with settling or litigating individual claims; these are primarily defense attorney and expert witness fees.
3. *Operating expenses* include all other expenses incurred by the insurance company. Such expenses include underwriting, claims administration, finance, computer systems, marketing, and agent commissions.

However, there are a number of areas in which insurance differs from other businesses. The most important area is the need to collect an appropriate amount of premium today to cover the cost of losses and legal defense that may, and often do, occur 4 to 6 years in the future. By definition, actual future costs are unknown at the time the insurer must price and sell the policy. If insurers seriously underestimate future costs and fall into insolvency, the physician is left without the liability protection that he or she paid for, but the liability remains. Therefore, the choice of a malpractice insurance company is an important one for physicians. The true value of a policy (as opposed to its cost) may not be apparent until years after the purchase, when a claim must be defended and possibly paid.

The following principles of insurance and definitions of key terms are intended to facilitate that choice.

SPREAD OF RISK

Physicians as a group, knowing some of them will be sued and will have to pay litigation costs and losses, pool resources to share the total burden of the group. In any given year, not every physician will be sued, but all will contribute to cover the costs of those who are. In return, the individual physician is protected in similar fashion when he or she is the target of litigation. By assembling a large enough group, the burden on any individual, even those faced with large claims, can be reduced. The law of large numbers puts prediction of outcomes on a more sound statistical footing.

UNDERWRITING

The insurance company reviews every physician applicant and divides the group into multiple subgroups that share similar risk profiles. Some of the attributes that significantly affect risk include the level of education and training, specialty, the state and county where the practice is located, nature of practice, unusual practice profiles, clinical setting, and previous litigation history. This means, for example, that a neurosurgeon in Florida will be asked to pay a very different premium than a pediatrician in California.

It doesn't have to be this way. In theory, the costs of litigation, expense, and profit could simply be added up and divided equally among all policyholders. However, that would mean that physicians at lower risk for claims would be subsidizing those at higher risk. To our knowledge, no company is currently organized along these lines.

Periodically, a prudent insurance carrier reviews each policyholder's experience to determine whether the risk profile has changed. This involves a review of the litigation experience, the practice profile, and any changes in medical, legal, or professional status (e.g., licensing actions or substance abuse problems). The purpose of this exercise is to be sure the premium burden continues to be equitably apportioned among the pool.

ACTUARIAL SCIENCE AND FINANCIAL MARKETS

Actuaries use a variety of complex mathematical models to estimate future loss and legal defense costs based on past experience, estimates of future trends in claims severity and frequency, and the anticipated composition of the risk pool. These models must reflect the impact of past and prospective changes in the economic (e.g., inflation) and legal (e.g., tort reform) environments. Because there is a long time gap from the collection of premiums to the closing of the average claim file, these models must also reflect the value of investment income. Part of the fiduciary responsibility of any insurance company is to responsibly invest premium until the money is needed to pay future losses and expenses. The investment income collected during that period can be used to subsidize the actual cost of premiums. For this reason, insurance rates are sensitive to the state of the investment markets, primarily interest rates. (The average malpractice insurer maintains 80–90% of its investment portfolio in investment grade bonds—not stocks). As interest rates rise or fall, the amount of money available to subsidize policyholder charges varies. In low-interest rate environments, premiums must more closely match costs. In higher return settings, insurers may be able to sell insurance for less than cost and still remain solvent.

CLAIMS MADE VS OCCURRENCE COVERAGE

Before the insurance crises of the 1970s, malpractice insurance was sold on an *occurrence* basis. Any claim arising from an event occurring in the policy period would be covered, regardless of when the claim was reported or when in the future it needed to be paid. This type of policy makes it difficult for insurance companies to predict the ultimate cost of losses, because today's premiums must cover future losses regardless of when they are reported. The mass litigation surrounding asbestos and toxic waste that is occurring presently, many decades after the insurance was priced and sold and sometimes even prior to the identification of the potential risk, illustrates the difficulty with sustaining the occurrence form of insurance. For this reason, since the late 1970s, the majority of medical malpractice insurance policies for physicians is sold on a *claims made* basis. This form requires that a covered event must occur and the claim must be made (reported) during the policy period. Claims made coverage can be extended back by adding *nose* coverage, in which the insurer agrees to cover claims made during the policy period based on events that occurred prior to the inception date of the policy. When a physician retires or chooses to move to a different insurance carrier, he or she may obtain *tail* coverage. This provides insurance for a covered event occurring during the policy period, even if the claim is not reported until later. In the case of a physician moving from one carrier to another, the individual can choose between tail coverage with the expiring carrier and nose coverage with the new carrier to accomplish the same purpose.

INCURRED LOSS AND RESERVES

Incurred loss represents the sum of losses actually paid plus a reserve for the costs of anticipated future losses. Loss reserves are both an estimate of the eventual cost of claims that are reported but still open and claims that have occurred and will be covered but have not yet been reported to the insurance company. The latter type of loss reserve is needed only for occurrence insurance and tail coverages.

As the claim for which a reserve is established closes, the final reserve, by definition, will match the actual cost of the claim. In addition, as more claims close and additional information on actual cost trends becomes known, the estimate of the ultimate cost of those claims that are still open may change. These changes are termed *development*. Reserve development can be up or down. If the ultimate cost of losses exceeds the original reserve estimate, the company would be said to be underreserved. If reserves exceed the actual cost of losses, the company would be said to be overreserved. In either case, the actual reserve figures must be adjusted as soon as available information warrants.

PROFIT OR LOSS

For most insurers, income is the sum of premium and investment income minus the cost of claims, underwriting, and other operating expenses. The *combined ratio* is defined as losses plus expenses divided by premium. It is a measure of the percentage of each premium dollar going to losses and expenses. A combined ratio of 100% means the company's claims losses and expenses exactly equal the premium collected. Insurance companies writing at a combined ratio of 100% would then have profit equal to investment income. Since the start of the recent crises beginning in 2000, the combined ratio of the average malpractice insurer has been between 130 and 140%, meaning that for every premium dollar collected, $1.40 is paid for losses and expenses. Obviously, such numbers produce very large operating losses even when investment income is included.

SURPLUS

An insurance company's assets minus its liabilities equal its surplus. This represents the capital base of the company and, in a mutual or reciprocal insurance company, belongs to the policyholders. It is necessary to maintain significant surplus to support company operations and to maintain solvency during those years when unpredictably high losses are incurred. Insurance companies are regulated by State Departments of Insurance that require certain amounts of surplus to back each dollar of premium and reserves. The intent is to provide assurance to policyholders that a company has sufficient assets to pay their claims, even if losses are greater than anticipated. Surplus is also needed to provide the capital backing necessary to accept new business.

REINSURANCE

Reinsurance is an agreement between insurance companies under which one company accepts all or part of the risk of the other. Most insurance companies insure only part of the risk assumed on any given policy. The amount of this primary layer of coverage varies among carriers. Smaller carriers may themselves cover the first $250,000 of loss, whereas larger companies may retain the first $1 million. The insurance company takes a portion of the premium collected from the policyholder and *cedes* it to the reinsurer to cover losses under clearly defined circumstances. This is the principle of spread of risk applied to insurance companies and is intended to mitigate the effect of very large losses on a single company. The less primary risk that the company retains, the more premium it has to pay to the reinsurer to cover the remaining policy limits. Thus, reinsurance is a necessary aspect of financial prudence for the vast majority of insurance companies; however, it ultimately adds cost (the reinsurer's profit or margin) in exchange for the protection it provides against unexpected or very large losses.

II   LEGAL

2

What Every Doctor Should Know About Litigation

A Primer on How to Win Medical Malpractice Lawsuits

Fred J. Hiestand, JD

SUMMARY

This chapter explains what you should know to best look out for yourself and how you should go about doing so. Its premise is that just as patients should not leave decisions about the best course of medical treatment exclusively to medical professionals, neither should you as a doctor or health care provider leave your fate as a defendant solely in the hands of your lawyer and insurer. No one representing you will be as affected as you are by the litigation in which you are a defendant; and, although your advocates are charged with looking after your best interests, your active and intelligent participation in how they do this is absolutely necessary if they are to be effective.

Key Words: Defendant; storyteller; discovery; duty; causation; negligence; reform; MICRA.

From: *Medical Malpractice: A Physician's Sourcebook*
Edited by: R. E. Anderson © Humana Press Inc., Totowa, NJ

INTRODUCTION: PURPOSE AND SCOPE

If you are a medical professional, chances are you will be sued during your career.[1] Whether named as a principal or peripheral defendant, once served with summons you or your professional liability insurer must pay for your defense and, should you lose or settle the case, for satisfaction of your liability. Understanding the essentials of litigation enables you to eliminate or at the very least minimize your liability and get on with your life. Not knowing this information leaves you with little or no control over your own destiny, a wisp to be buffeted about by the devil's breath of litigation.

This chapter explains what you should know to best look out for yourself and how you should go about doing so. Its premise is that just as patients should not leave decisions about the best course of medical treatment exclusively to medical professionals, neither should you as a doctor or health care provider leave your fate as a defendant solely in the hands of your lawyer and insurer. No one representing you will be as affected as you are by the litigation in which you are a defendant; and, although your advocates are charged with looking after your best interests, your active and intelligent participation in how they do this is absolutely necessary if they are to be effective. Most understand that "knowledge is power." We can also appreciate that sometimes, as the cliché goes, a little knowledge may be a dangerous thing. However, the information given here can—if properly digested—make your life safer and more secure from the slings and arrows of outrageous lawsuits.

---

[1] "No doctor is safe from Trial Lawyers, Inc. A 2002 *Medical Economics* survey of 1800 physicians found that 58% had been the target of a lawsuit." (*Trial Lawyers Inc—A Report on the Lawsuit Industry in America 2003*, Center for Legal Policy, The Manhattan Inst., 2003, p. 12); "The first medical malpractice suit in the United States was brought in 1794. However, it was not until the 1930's that the number of claims against doctors began to significantly increase. Medical malpractice claims continued to become more common in U.S. courts until reaching a peak in the 1970's, when there were so many claims that chaos ensued. It was said that there were approximately 'five malpractice suits filed annually for every 10 doctors.'" (Jason Leo, Note: *Torts – Medical Malpractice: The Legislature's Attempt to Prevent Cases Without Merit Denies Valid Claims* (2000) 27 *Wm. Mitchell L. Rev.* 1399, 1402–1403); "Prior to 1960, only one in seven physicians had been sued in their entire career; presently claims are filed against one out of seven physicians per annum." (Rima J. Oken, *Note: Curing Healthcare Providers' Failure to Administer Opioids in the Treatment of Severe Pain* (2002) 23 *Cardozo L. Rev.* 1917, 1968, fn. 252).

Why This Chapter Can Help You

"The life of the law," Oliver Wendell Holmes said, "has not been logic; it has been experience."[2]

This chapter is derived from the litigation experiences of a seasoned practitioner. The first 3 years of my civil legal practice was in poverty law representing farm workers and senior citizens; the next 3 years in public interest law for various clients, including prisoners, senior citizen organizations, and the Black Panther Party. In the three decades since then, I have had my own civil practice representing numerous clients in various matters, including the defense of doctors and other health care providers in malpractice cases. A significant portion of this work has been in the trial courts, although most of it comes from working on appeals in California state and federal courts. Some of what is shared here also comes from consulting for the California Legislature and former Governor Jerry Brown on medical liability reform legislation, specifically the law known as the Medical Liability Reform Act (MICRA). Since MICRA's enactment in 1975, I have continued to represent health care providers in the courts and as a legislative advocate to preserve and protect it from erosion or repeal.

Appellate practice focuses on what happens after a judgment or ruling in a lower court from which a dissatisfied party seeks reversal in a higher court. An appellate lawyer has a vantage point analogous to that of an historian: he or she must sift through the record of proceedings in the court below looking for legal or evidentiary error to determine if reversal is warranted. This quarrying gives the appellate advocate a grasp on what can and does go wrong and right in litigation and enables one to discern from these case histories what should and should not be done to win in liability disputes. Legislative advocacy complements appellate practice by adding a public policy dimension to the issues that constantly recur in medical liability disputes. It is from this trove of litigation and legislative experience that this chapter is composed. Emphasis is on California law, although reference also is made to comparable laws in other states; however, the objective is less to understand the details of the rules than the dynamic interplay between them that can and does occur when you try to navigate the rough shoals of litigation.

---

[2] O.W. Holmes, Jr. *The Mind and Faith of Justice Holmes 51* (M. Lerner, ed. 1943).

Mastering Litigation Rules and Honing Storytelling Skills: The Keys to Winning Lawsuits

The overall approach or perspective a party to a lawsuit should have to win or best survive it is twofold: that of a game player and storyteller. The game[3] played is, to be sure, a high stakes one in which you can affect the outcome to win, lose, or draw (i.e., settle). To my mind, "winning" in the context of malpractice litigation means getting out of it as early as possible with no judgment of liability against you. If you have to go to trial, even if you eventually win your case, you will pay such a heavy price that the victory will seem pyrrhic. That is because preparing for trial, let alone going through it, is a lengthy and arduous process that consumes your time and physical and emotional resources to the neglect of your present and future life. In preparing for trial, you will be forced to put much of your present life on hold while you concentrate on reliving an event that happened in the past, frequently several years in the past. Dwelling on the past in a defensive way prevents you from realizing the present and planning for the future; it is by all accounts a draining process.[4] Therefore, your objective, and that of the team defending you, must be to rid yourself of the Damoclean lawsuit at the earliest opportunity.

The storytelling aspect of litigation requires your defense team to put a consistent "spin" or interpretation on the known and unknown facts that is a more persuasive explanation of what happened than the interpretation provided by the plaintiff. These "facts" will emerge in varying degrees of clarity from medical records and witness testi-

---

[3] Use of the term "game" is not meant to trivialize or minimize the importance of the litigation process, but rather to get the reader to better understand how to maneuver within it by "seeing" it in the sense that Wittgenstein sees what all games share: "You will not see something that is common to *all,* but similarities, relationships and a whole series of them at that." (Ludwig Wittgenstein, *Philosophical Investigations*, 3rd Ed., 1968, § 66 [emphasis original].) Wittgenstein refers to this network of interrelatedness as "family resemblances." (*Id.* § 67.)

[4] "According to a Harvard University study, about 20 percent of doctors who are sued for malpractice rate this event as the most significant in their life. Additionally, 40 percent undergo a major depression as a result and 60 percent state that being sued for malpractice has altered their lives and practices completely." Richard Vinson, MD, *Blame Lawsuits*, Letter-to-the Editor, *El Paso Times*, El Paso, Texas: May 21, 2002, p. 6A.

mony, but they must be constantly placed in a context that will make sense to those deciding your case. This presupposes that although much can be learned about what happened to someone else in the course of medical treatment that is related to some injury that befalls the plaintiff, there will invariably be ambiguity about many aspects of what is learned. The longer litigation persists and the closer it gets to trial, the more facts will be known to both sides that require explanation as to why they do or do not add up to the defendant's liability. Ultimately, if one must go to trial, the audience that hears and judges what is the best or most credible story will be the court and jury or arbitrator(s).

Whatever attempts are made along the way to dispose of the case before trial will require a nonfiction narrative that is more believable than your opponent's story, that makes better sense of what is known and not known factually than a contrary explanation pointing to your liability. Stories you tell along the way to trial must be consistent with each other even if the latest spin is, as expected, more detailed than earlier versions you present. Conflicting stories or interpretations of facts will, if they are known to court or jury, hurt your credibility and increase the risk of a finding of liability against you.

With this sketch of the big litigation picture in mind, let us turn to rules of the game and then discuss what you should do from the time you are first forced to play the game.

THE IMPORTANCE OF THE RULES
IN THE LITIGATION GAME

To win or avoid losing in any game other than one of pure chance, a player must be generally familiar with the rules of that game and the moves, likely and actual, of other players in it. That familiarity should not be on the detailed nuances of the rules, which is the responsibility of your lawyers, but on the importance and dynamics of the interplay between them. Rules of litigation fall into three categories: substantive, procedural, and evidentiary.

The Substantive Liability Rule of Negligence
and Its Four Constituent Elements of Duty,
Breach, Causation, and Compensable Injury

Substantive rules are those that define the conditions necessary to find liability. When it comes to professional liability or medical malpractice, the most common substantive rule is *negligence*. Negligence is comprised of four essential elements, and the absence of any one element defeats liability. The first element is that a defendant must be shown to owe a *duty* to the plaintiff. This means that there must be a defined and accepted standard of care that the defendant is required to adhere to in treating the plaintiff, something the defendant should not have done that he or she did or some act that he or she did that should not have been done. Standards of care can be found in statutes, regulations, court decisions, published professional articles, and testimony by expert medical witnesses. When the standard of care is a statute, regulation, or rule of a professional organization, its violation is called *negligence per se.*

The second element that must be proved to successfully prosecute a medical malpractice case is that the defendant *breached* this standard of care, which is to say that he or she acted contrary to or in violation of it. This is usually an evidentiary matter where each side presents whatever testimony or documentary evidence that shows conduct by the defendant in conformity with or in violation of the standard of care. Where there is a conflict in the evidence about breach, the factfinder—most commonly a jury—must decide whether the evidence presented favors the plaintiff or defendant on this point.

Third, it must be proved that the defendant's breach of the duty of care owed to the plaintiff caused the plaintiff injury. Causation is of two kinds: factual and legal. Not surprisingly, factual causation is determined by the factfinder or jury, unless the case is before a judge acting by stipulation as the factfinder or by an arbitrator. The test for *factual causation*, what was once called "but for" causation, is whether the breach was a substantial factor in bringing about injury to the plaintiff. However, *legal causation*, what the law used to call proximate cause, is a policy or scope of liability determination made by the court or judge. It is an aspect of negligence liability in which courts address whether they are going to draw a "bright line," beyond which they will not impose liability as a matter of law even if the conduct at issue is deemed factually responsible for the plaintiff's injury.

Finally, as already implied, a plaintiff must prove that satisfaction of all the foregoing elements resulted in his *compensable injury.* In other words, a plaintiff must prove that his or her injuries are of a nature that may be redressed by monetary damages. Damages are of two principal kinds: economic and noneconomic. *Economic loss* is damage that can be objectively measured like lost wages and medical care, both past and future. *Noneconomic damage* is subjective and immeasurable, like pain and suffering or loss of consortium (i.e., companionship).

Procedural and Evidentiary Rules

Procedural rules determine how and when the substantive rules do or do not come into play and how information is gathered that bears on the substantive rules. Finding information that may include or lead to admissible evidence is done through the procedural rules of discovery. The most common procedural rules of discovery include written interrogatories, requests for admission, requests to produce documents, oral depositions, and requests for designation of experts. Procedural rules that can terminate litigation or alter its focus are the subject of law and motion practice.

Evidentiary rules determine what facts get considered or precluded from consideration by the court, jury, or arbitrators to determine whether the substantive conditions of liability are satisfied. These rules determine what testimony, documents, photographs, recordings, and the like are admissible and what weight should be given to particular evidence admitted.

How Medical Malpractice Reform Changes the Conventional Rules of the Litigation Game

Numerous states faced with malpractice insurance crises over the past 30 years have made changes to their litigation rules—substantive, procedural, and evidentiary—in an attempt to cabin the number of lawsuits and the size of awards to better protect the public's access to uninterrupted health care. In 1975, California was the first state to do this in a significant way when it enacted MICRA in response to the medical malpractice insurance crisis the state was then undergoing and has since avoided repeating. MICRA exists to reduce the cost and increase the efficiency of medical malpractice litigation by revising numerous legal rules applicable to such litigation. This comprehensive reform package illustrates how changes in all three categories of litigation rules can produce stability and certainty in the determination of who gets how much, from whom, and under what circumstances when someone is injured in the course of medical treatment and seeks redress.

MICRA's success in accomplishing its stated purpose has made it a model for states experiencing problems in assuring continued access to health care stemming from an unstable litigation and liability insurance climate; it is also a model for federal legislation endorsed by the President George W. Bush and the House of Representatives but thus far blocked from enactment by a lack of support in the US Senate.

THE LIMITATIONS ON RECOVERABLE NONECONOMIC DAMAGE, PLAINTIFF
LAWYER'S CONTINGENCY FEES, AND THE STATUTE OF LIMITATIONS

One change made to the substantive liability rule of negligence by
MICRA was with respect to the amount recoverable in noneconomic
damages by a plaintiff. That amount is capped at $250,000.[5] Other
states have comparable limits, most restricting this category of damage somewhere between $250,000 and $400,000. This ceiling on a
subjective, immeasurable component of recoverable damage is the
heart of MICRA and the provision most vexing to personal injury
lawyers who traditionally relied on these damages to cover their attorney fees.[6] There is an impressive body of authority showing that the
nonpecuniary damage ceiling has been particularly effective in arrest-
ing spiraling awards and stabilizing medical liability insurance rates.

Another reform in MICRA is the sliding contingency fee scale for
plaintiff attorneys, which assures that the greater a plaintiff's injuries
and damages, the larger the percentage of the total award that goes to
the plaintiff, with a corresponding reduced share to the plaintiff's lawyer. As a report of an American Bar Association commission explained
long ago about this kind of provision: "[In] order to relate the attorney's
fee more to the amount of legal work and expense involved in handling
a case and less to the fortuity of the plaintiff's economic status and
degree of injury, a decreasing maximum schedule of attorney's fees,
reasonably generous in the lower recovery ranges and thus unlikely to
deny potential plaintiffs access to legal representation, should be set on
a state-by-state basis."[7]

A third medical liability reform in MICRA and other state statutes
that may be considered substantive, because it undeniably affects the
outcome of many claims, is the shortening and tightening of the statute
of limitations for medical malpractice claims.[8] The *limitations period*

---

[5] Ca. Civ. C. § 3333.2.

[6] "Awards for pain and suffering serve to ease plaintiffs' discomfort and to
pay for attorney fees for which plaintiffs are not otherwise compensated."
Seffert v. Los Angeles Transit Lines, 1961 56 Cal.2d 498, 511 (dissenting
opinion by Traynor, J.).

[7] *Rep. of Com. on Medical Professional Liability* (1977) 102 ABA Annual
Rep. 786, 851. *See also* Dept. of HEW, *Rep. of Sect's. Com. on Medical Malpractice* (1973) pp. 34–35.

[8] Cal. Code of Civ. Proc. § 340.5.

is the time during which a suit must be filed after the injury occurs or, absent an express waiver by the defendant, it is barred. Before MICRA and analogous statutes in other states, the limitations period was practically open-ended, making stale claims common and resulting in a "long-tail" for liability that prevented accurate claims forecasting and predictable premium setting.[9]

REFORM OF THE COLLATERAL SOURCE RULE

Traditionally, when an injured plaintiff gets some compensation for the injury from a collateral source such as health, life, or disability insurance, that payment, under the collateral source doctrine, is not deducted from the damages that the plaintiff can collect from the defendant.[10] The collateral source rule is "generally accepted in the United States"[11] and implemented by barring the factfinder from hearing any evidence about collateral source benefits. Underlying this rule is the public policy rationale that it "encourage[s] citizens to purchase and maintain insurance for personal injuries and for other eventualities... If we were to permit [defendants] to mitigate damages with payments from plaintiff's insurance, plaintiff would be in a position inferior to that of having bought no insurance, because his payment of premiums would have earned no benefit. Defendant should not be able to avoid payment of full compensation for the injury inflicted merely because the victim has had the foresight to provide himself with insurance."[12]

MICRA alters this evidentiary rule in medical malpractice cases by specifying that a medical malpractice defendant may introduce evidence of collateral source benefits received by or payable to the plaintiff. When a defendant chooses to introduce such evidence, the plaintiff may introduce evidence of the amounts he or she has paid, for example,

---

[9] "More than a decade may pass before a suit is brought on an incident involving a minor. This further complicates the methods of establishing rates, and is inequitable since the vast majority of medial malpractice committed on infants is detectable within the normal statute of limitations." California Assembly Select Committee on Medical Malpractice, *Preliminary Report* (1974), p. 10.

[10] See 1 Dobbs, *Law of Remedies*, 2nd Ed., 1993, § 3.8(1), pp. 372–373.

[11] *Helfend v. Southern Cal. Rapid Transit Dist.* (1970) 2 Cal.3d 1; *see also* *Rest.2d Torts*, §§ 920, 920A.

[12] *Helfend, supra*, 2 Cal.3d at 10 .

in insurance premiums,– to secure the benefits. Although this modification of the collateral source rule does not specify how the jury should use such evidence, the underlying legislative presumption and the practical effect is that in most cases, the jury sets plaintiff damages at a lower level because of its awareness of plaintiff net collateral source benefits. Other states have altered their collateral source for medical negligence cases to explicitly mandate a deduction of the amount of the collateral sources from the plaintiff's award.[13]

Courts repelling constitutional challenges to MICRA like collateral source reforms recognize that alteration of this conventional evidentiary bar leads to lower malpractice awards and directly relates to the objective of reducing the costs incurred by malpractice defendants and their insurers. Reputable studies confirm the correctness of this conclusion.[14] As the California Supreme Court remarked, "The Legislature could reasonably have determined that the reduction of such costs would serve the public interest by preserving the availability of medical care throughout the state and by helping to assure that patients who were injured by medical malpractice in the future would have a source of medical liability insurance to cover their losses."[15] Indeed, in analyzing the collateral source rule, the Court acknowledged that most legal commentators had severely criticized it for affording a plaintiff a double recovery for losses not really sustained and noted that "many jurisdictions had either restricted or repealed it."[16]

ALTERATION OF THE "LUMP SUM" JUDGMENT RULE

At common law, a plaintiff who suffers bodily injury at the hands of a tortfeasor has traditionally been compensated for both past and

---

[13] See Comment, *An Analysis of State Legislative Responses to the Medical Malpractice Crisis Duke L.J.* 1975;1417:1447–1450.

[14] See Patricia M. Danzon, *The Frequency and Severity of Medical Malpractice Claims: New Evidence, Law & Contemp. Probs.*, Spring 1986, at 57, 72 (collateral source offset associated with 14% decrease in claim frequency); *id.* at 77 (collateral source offset associated with decrease in amount of awards by 11 to 18%).

[15] *Fein v. Permanente Medical Group* (1985) 38 Cal.3d 137, 166.

[16] *Helfend v. Southern Cal. Rapid Transit District, supra,* 2 Cal.3d at 13.

future damages through a "lump sum" judgment, payable at the conclusion of the trial.[17] However, increasingly in the past half century, tort scholars have recognized that lump sum awards often are dissipated by improvident expenditures or investments before the injured person actually incurs the future medical expenses or earning losses. Accordingly, they have advocated legislative adoption of a "periodic payment" procedure as a reform measure that would, in these commentators' view, benefit both plaintiffs and defendants.[18] Many states have responded with statutes authorizing the periodic payment of damages in various tort fields,[19] especially medical malpractice. These statutory reforms are classic procedural laws.

---

[17] 2 Harper & James, *The Law of Torts* (1956) § 25.2, p. 1303.

[18] See *id.*, at pp. 1303–1304; Keeton & O'Connell, *Basic Protection for the Traffic Victim—A Blueprint for Reforming Automobile Insurance* (1965) pp. 351–358; Henderson, *Periodic Payments of Bodily Injury Awards* (1980) 66 *A.B.A.J.* 734.

[19] See, for example, Ala. Code § 6-11-3(3) (future damages of more than $150,000 to be paid periodically); Alaska Stat. § 09.17.040(d) (periodic payment judgment mandated if requested by injured party); Cal. Code of Civ. P. § 667.7 (periodic payment judgment mandated if requested by any party to a medical malpractice action and the award for future damages is at least $50,000); Fla. Stat. § 766.209(4)(a) (periodic payment judgment mandated if requested by medical malpractice defendant whose offer of binding arbitration was refused by the claimant), § 768.78(1) (periodic payment judgment permitted if requested by any party); Kan. Stat. Ann. § 603407(c)(3) (judgment in medical malpractice action in the form of an annuity to be entered for future economic damages if noneconomic and accrued economic damages award do not exceed overall cap); Md. Code Ann., Cts. & Jud. Proc. § 11-109(c)(1) (periodic payments listed as a permitted alternative form for future economic damages in medical malpractice actions); N.H. Rev. Stat. Ann. § 507-C:7 IV (in action for "medical injury" periodic payment of future damages permitted if amount greater than $50,000 and any party so requests); N.M. Stat. Ann. § 41-5-7(D) (future medical and related care damages from medical malpractice to be paid as expenses incurred); S.D. Codified Laws Ann. § 21-3A-2 (periodic payment judgment permitted if requested by any party to a medical malpractice action); Utah Code Ann. § 78-14-9.5 (periodic payment of future damages required if requested by any party); Wash. Rev. Code § 4.56.260 (at a party's request, any award for future economic damages of at least $100,000 to be entered as a periodic payment judgment).

Legislatures that have enacted periodic payment laws for future damages concluded that this will further the fundamental goal of matching losses with compensation by helping to ensure that money paid to an injured plaintiff will, in fact, be available when the plaintiff incurs the anticipated expenses or losses in the future. In addition, they determined that the public interest is served by limiting a defendant's obligation to those future damages that a plaintiff actually incurs, eliminating windfalls obtained by a plaintiff's heirs when they inherit a portion of a lump sum judgment that was intended to compensate the injured person for losses he never sustained. As the California Supreme Court stated when, against constitutional attack, it upheld that state's periodic payment provision:[20]

> One of the factors which contributed to the high cost of malpractice insurance was the need for insurance companies to retain large reserves to pay out sizeable lump sum awards. The adoption of a periodic payment procedure permits insurers to retain fewer liquid reserves and to increase investments, thereby reducing the costs to insurers and, in turn, to insureds. In addition, the portion of [the periodic payment statute] which provides for the termination of a significant portion of the remaining future damage payments in the event of the plaintiff's death is obviously related to the goal of reducing insurance costs.

HOW THE VARIOUS RULES "FIT" WITHIN THE LEGAL HIERARCHY

Notice that most of the rules discussed so far are state *statutes* or judge-made by courts where the liability disputes arise. Court- or judge-made rules (they are synonymous) are known as *common law* rules. They are derived from particular factual disputes and, after articulation of them by the court as a guiding principle for future cases, have the force of *stare decisis* or precedent. Precedent is to be followed by future courts unless it is has outlived its usefulness or no longer makes sense. That decision is made by an intermediate appellate court or the highest court in that state or by the legislature. When the defendant in a professional liability case is the federal government or its employees, or arises under particularly defined circumstances that implicate federal law,

---

[20]*American Bank & Trust Co. v. Superior Court* 36 Cal.3d 1984;359, 372,373.

then federal courts decide the dispute according to federal statutes and federal common law.

All statutes—federal and state—must be interpreted or applied by courts to particular facts. This naturally gives courts some leeway to clarify the application of the statute and, by so doing, put an additional gloss on its plain language. If a statute is itself a statement of the common law, there is authority that a court can just amend it by interpreting it in light of changing circumstances and conditions. When statues are amended in ways a legislature does not like, it can "correct" the court's interpretation by restating or further amending the statute. In interpreting statutes courts must look to pertinent constitutional provisions, the *purpose* of the statute, how it relates to other statutes that also apply to the dispute, and to *canons of statutory interpretation* or aids in reading the text and ascertaining whether the enacting body "said what it meant, and meant what it said."

Sometimes a statute is challenged for its validity, either on its face or as applied, by reference to the federal and applicable state *constitutions.* A federal statute cannot be invalidated on constitutional grounds except by reference to the US Constitution. A state statute, however, must comply with *both* the federal and state constitutions as well as with federal statutory law that preempts the field. Although generally a statute found in compliance with the US Constitution also satisfies its corresponding state constitutional cognate, this is not always so. State constitutions sometimes provide *greater* protection to their citizens than analogous provisions of the federal constitution.

The interplay between the hierarchy of courts and related statutes and constitutional provisions is an important dynamic to keep in mind when playing the litigation game. For example, from 1872 to 1975, California personal injury cases were governed by the rule of contributory negligence, a rule that by popular consensus was embodied in a statute unchanged in wording from when originally enacted.[21] *Contributory negligence* means that if a defendant could show that the plaintiff's own negligence contributed to his or her injury, even to a small degree, then the plaintiff is completely barred from any recovery

---

[21] "Everyone is responsible, not only for the result of his willful acts, but also for an injury occasioned to another by his want of ordinary care or skill in the management of his property or person, *except so far as the latter has, willfully or by want of ordinary care, brought the injury upon himself.*" (Cal. Civ. C. § 1714; italics added.)

against the defendant. Yet when that statute was challenged as unfair in *Li v. Yellow Cab Co.*,[22] California's supreme court agreed and interpreted it as suddenly providing, *mutatis mutandis*, for *comparative negligence*: This means that the assessment of liability in California and the majority of states that have since adopted comparative fault in place of contributory fault is based on the plaintiff's proportionate share of fault to the total universe of negligence; so that a plaintiff 25% negligent for his or her own injuries should only have damages reduced by that percent of the total loss incurred, not be barred entirely from recovery.

Another illustration of how the dynamic interplay between the rules of procedure, evidence and substantive liability can dispose of a malpractice case short of trial is *Martinez v. Ha, M.D.* [23] An orthopedic surgeon performed a complete knee replacement on the plaintiff, who developed a serious infection shortly afterward that necessitated a knee fusion. The plaintiff sued claiming that the doctor had not washed his hands and caused the infection. The doctor moved to summarily dispose of the case, presenting expert written testimony that there was no evidence he had caused the infection in plaintiff's knee. Plaintiff opposed the motion, but did not submit any expert testimony contradicting the doctor; so the court ruled for the doctor. On appeal judgment was affirmed, the appellate court stating that the lower "court was presented with uncontroverted evidence that [plaintiff] could not prove at least one element [i.e., causation] of his claim." [24]

What *Li* and *Martinez* underscore is that a successful litigator must always be aware of the dynamic interplay of the rules and of new interpretations of them that can yield different results from the old readings.

The Importance of the Players
in the Litigation Game and of Storytelling

The players include the parties, their attorneys, witnesses, and the court and jury (or in some cases, arbitrators). The players who are parties to the litigation (i.e., plaintiffs and defendants) can voluntarily agree to end the game at any time, which is the outcome of most litigation; however, this only occurs when they have assessed that the consequences

---

[22] (1975) 13 C.3d 804.

[23] 12 P.3d 1159 (2000 Alas.).

[24] Id. at 1163.

of continuing it are likely riskier in terms of their self-interest than capping it. That assessment is an ongoing one based on the progress of the game and how application of the rules and the moves by the players stack up at any given time.

The Lawyers

Lawyers are indispensable to lawsuits. Indeed, they are so essential that a popular saw holds that "any town that won't support one lawyer, will always support two." They are the legal representatives of their clients, which means they speak for them to the universe concerned about your dispute. If the lawyer makes a bad impression on others in that universe it hurts the client. It is largely through lawyers that the court and jury will assess you and your adversary, and determine who to favor in various decisions. Lawyers are, in essence, the main strategists and tellers of their clients' stories. Your lawyer is also your guide through the legal labyrinth you must traverse; it is by and through your lawyer that, if you ask the right questions, you will learn the options available to win your case. You need and deserve the best lawyer you can get for your case.

Defendants in medical malpractice cases typically turn to their liability insurance company for a lawyer. Usually the carriers can be counted on to provide those they insure with well-qualified attorneys because they share with them the objective of winning. When the carrier informs you about the lawyer or law firm they have in mind to defend you, ask for a resume of the lawyer. Pick up the telephone if the lawyer has not contacted you first, and have a frank discussion about the attorney's qualifications and experience. How long has the lawyer been in practice? How many medical malpractice cases has he litigated? What have been the results? Does he know the plaintiff's attorney? Has he ever been on the opposite side of a case against the plaintiff's attorney and, if so, what happened? Check standard news sources, jury verdicts, and databases of appellate cases to see what you can learn about the attorney.

Occasionally, the chemistry between a client and counsel is not good. If that should happen to you, if you don't have a comfortable or confident feeling about your prospective or assigned attorney after conferring with him or her, be honest. A good lawyer understands the importance of a positive attorney–client relationship, as does you malpractice insurer. Trust and confidence are the cornerstones to this, every bit as much as they are essential to the physician–patient relationship.

Regrettably, people who would not hesitate to grill a contractor for a prospective home remodel about past projects and references, become shy when it comes to selecting counsel for representation that could affect their careers. Don't make that mistake; it is much more difficult to switch lawyers in the middle of litigation because of a bad initial selection than it is to take the time to be as reasonably sure as you can be that you have chosen the best person to represent you. Martindale-Hubbell is a quick source of basic biographical information about lawyers. Newspaper articles and electronic databases of information mentioning the lawyers involved in published opinions and jury verdicts are other sources of useful information.

You are not required to accept whatever attorney is recommended to you, no more than your carrier is required to accept and pay for any attorney you may like but who knows little or nothing about medical malpractice. You and your professional liability insurer should, because you have the same interest in achieving the most favorable outcome for you, be able to agree on a good attorney, one with the education and experience best suited for your needs.

"Here Comes the Judge!"

Judges are the principal representatives of the court; they interpret and apply the law and, when a jury is involved, instruct it on the applicable legal rules. Although a jury is usually involved in a medical malpractice case, courts can, by agreement of the parties, sit as both the "finder" of facts and law. An arbitrator or panel of arbitrators, of course, act as determiners of both the law and facts. Judges and arbitrators also rule on motions that can dispose of or shape the course of the litigation and rule on what evidence is admissible. Obviously, who one gets for a judge can be critical to the case, so it's important to know as much as one can about the judge or arbitrator who will hear the case. The best source of information about judges and arbitrators is, not surprisingly, other lawyers who have tried cases before them. Because most defense attorneys practice primarily where they live, they will know about the judge or at least know someone else who has tried cases before, or knows the judge. Certain public information is also available about judges, including information about cases on which they have decided or ruled. From these varied sources, one can usually discover whether a judge has a reputation for fairness, knowledge of the law, is intellectually bright or slow, and has a quick or even temper.

Many, if not all, states permit one peremptory challenge to a judge and all allow a challenge based on bias. It is common in larger urban areas to assign a different judge for pretrial motions from the judge drawn for settlement discussion and trial, so research on the universe of judges one is likely to draw for each of these stages of litigation is advisable.

The Jury

Jurors decide factual disputes, which means that they determine the ultimate "facts" of your case. Their judgment as to what the "facts" are, including the fact and size of damages should they decide to award them, cannot be disturbed on appeal unless it can be shown that there is no substantial evidence to support those findings. When a judge or arbitrator also acts as the "fact finder," this same restrained standard of review—"substantial evidence"—also applies.

Selection of jurors naturally comes just before the case is to be tried, which means that the parties will have gathered all their evidence and should be ready for trial. Each party, through counsel, will have some opportunity to question or submit questions to the judge to ask of each juror. The law refers to this as the *voir dire* of prospective jurors. Usually, each party has a limited number of peremptory challenges and may also challenge a juror for "good cause" or bias, on which the judge will rule.

Some lawyers are fond of employing, for big cases, jury consultants, professional "jury experts" who read body language and pay particular attention to the responses jurors make to the *voir dire* questions. Other lawyers trust their own instincts when it comes to accepting or challenging certain jurors; and some even feel that it doesn't matter in the end which jurors are selected; they take any panel that meets with the judge's approval. If your case looks like it is going to trial and you feel you have a good sense of people, your lawyer should be willing to listen to you in the jury selection process.

Witnesses, Especially "Experts"

All witnesses are important, especially you. This means witnesses should be well prepared. A prepared witness is not a "coached" witness; a "prepared" witness is one who understands the purpose for which his or her testimony is sought, and has some understanding of the questions likely to be asked. This requires a witness to think about the best and most honest way to respond to these questions. Your attorney will be able to and should prepare your witnesses. As for adversarial witnesses, pretrial discovery will reveal who they are and what they are likely to say and not say. Knowing this information will enable you and your attorney to fashion questions that show whether a witness is credible or, if credible, why mistaken about some key fact.

As a practical matter, in medical malpractice cases the most frequent source for defining the standard of care, as well as for determining the presence of other elements in the negligence calculus, is the *expert* witness. Who qualifies as an "expert" is defined by the law of the jurisdiction where the case is litigated. California, for example, which is typical of many jurisdictions, defines an expert as one who has "special knowledge, skill, experience, training or education" about the subject to which the testimony will relate.[25] Whether expert testimony is *admissible* (i.e., can be considered by the "fact finder") also depends on where the case is tried. Federal law, for instance, makes judges the "gate-keepers" for ensuring that scientific evidence is admitted *only* if it is both *relevant* and *reliable*.[26] Most significantly, the court must determine if the expert testimony offered has an adequate foundation, which means a judge has an independent duty to screen evidence and assure that it has a *rationally reliable basis*. In determining this, a court can consider whether the expert used the scientific method, whether the theory or technique relied upon has been subjected to peer review and publication, whether a particular scientific technique has a significant rate of error, and whether the methodology used is generally accepted in the relevant scientific community.

Medical malpractice cases are "expert driven." Experts are, as a general matter, best retained early to obtain their input on discovery and to aid in pretrial motions that can terminate or pare down issues in the case. Usually your attorney will want to retain a prospective expert in a given field as a "consultant" to the attorney; that way it will not be necessary to disclose your "expert's" identity and opinion on a matter should you decide not to use him or her as an "expert." The opinion would then be protected under the "work product" privilege of your attorney. If you or your adversary decide to go ahead with certain experts at trial, however, their identities must be disclosed by a certain time in the litigation framework to give each of you an opportunity to question the expert on his or her opinion before trial.

Although it used to be that the standard of care pertinent to medical negligence was a *local* one, the standard of care for sometime now has been a *national* one, which opens the door for both sides obtaining the "best" experts in the country. Moreover, because medicine is a dynamic and fast-changing profession, what was good medical practice yester-

---

[25] Cal. Evid. C. § 720(a); *Brown v. Colm* (1974) 11 Cal.3d 639.

[26] *Daubert v. Merrell Dow Pharmaceuticals, Inc.*, 509 U.S. 579, 587 (1993).

day may no longer be the case now; and an "expert" must be up on current medical advances and standards of care. The personal injury bar used to complain of a "conspiracy of silence," a tacit agreement amongst or common reluctance by doctors not to testify against their colleagues in medical negligence cases. Whatever truth there may have been to this accusation, a quick glance of the copious advertisements for "forensic medical experts" in the pages of magazines published by and for the personal injury bar shows that this is no longer true.

WHY IT IS CRITICALLY IMPORTANT TO "SEIZE THE TIME" WHEN SUED

Time can be critical to the outcome of litigation, a fact underscored by the often used legal phrase that "time is of the essence." The law provides that from the moment you are served with summons, the clock starts running on when you must respond to it and what devices will be available to you for that response. Usually, the period for filing an answer or other response is 30 days, a window by which, if your attorney acts promptly and intelligently, can give you a decided advantage over your adversary. If you waste or allow any of this time to pass in the belief (indisputably true) that you don't have to respond until the end of that 30 days, or that your attorney can probably get an extension of time by which to respond (almost always true), you could lose valuable opportunities to seize important advantages.

The Importance of Time in the Discovery Process

To illustrate the importance of time in litigation, consider the procedural device of discovery, the means by which parties are to find out from each other what evidence is known to that party or others in support or derogation of the lawsuit. One of these discovery mechanisms is the right to compel a party to appear and answer relevant questions under oath from your lawyer. This is called an *oral deposition*. The answers given to these questions often reveal facts that will determine whether the plaintiff has a viable claim against you or whether you have a defense against liability. Absent a showing to the court of "good cause," a plaintiff must normally wait 20 days after serving summons before noticing the defendant's deposition; however, the defendant need not wait any period of time after being served to notice the plaintiff's deposition.[27]

---

[27] Cal. Code of Civ. Proc. § 2025(b)(2).

A defendant has no waiting time other than the notice that must be given the plaintiff to appear for the deposition, usually 10 days, unless there is an order from the court shortening this time. Hence, it is possible for a defendant to get the jump on the plaintiff and smoke out his or her case early regarding the extent of damage suffered and why the plaintiff believes the defendant is responsible for it.

The longer you wait to take the plaintiff's deposition, the greater the likelihood that "facts" will be revealed or become "known" to the plaintiff that strengthen his or her case. For this reason, some defense lawyers prefer to wait to take the plaintiff's deposition until later in the lawsuit, especially because you usually only get one opportunity to take the plaintiff's deposition, unless there are unusual circumstances involved. However, if you have reason to believe the plaintiff has not put together a case by the time you are served, then it may be possible to get rid of the case early by showing that it is missing one or more elements critical to the liability equation.

Time and Summary Judgment or Summary Adjudication

Another procedural mechanism that can be combined with the prompt taking of the plaintiff's deposition is a *motion for summary judgment* or *partial summary adjudication*. This motion is a way for the court to look behind the pleadings and determine if the opposing party's pleadings lack evidentiary support that warrants limiting or terminating the lawsuit.[28] This is a particularly effective device for getting rid of a lawsuit where one of the essential elements of the substantive rules of liability is lacking; however, a defendant cannot invoke it earlier than 60 days after the complaint is filed, must give the plaintiff 75 days notice before it can be heard, and cannot have it heard later than 30 days before the date set for trial.[29] As a practical matter, these time requirements impose on defense counsel a burden to conduct sufficient discovery and investigation to put together the motion and file and serve it on the plaintiff 3.5 months before the date set for trial. A defendant who does not pay close attention to the passage of time could, through inadvertence, lose the right to invoke summary judgment and end up having to go to trial (perhaps unnecessarily).

---

[28] *Aguilar v. Atlantic Richfield Co.* (2001) 25 Cal.4th 826, 843.

[29] Cal. Code of Civ. Procedure § 437c(a); *McMahon v. Superior Court (American Equity Ins. Co.)* (2003) 106 Cal.App.4th 112, 116.

Therefore, when served with summons, you should immediately notify your medical liability insurer and get a copy of the summons and complaint to the appropriate representative. While doing this, you should also request your insurer to inform you right away of the lawyer who will be defending you. Do not wait for the lawyer to contact you. Once you know the identity of your counsel, contact him or her and ask to meet and confer about your case, preferably in person; however, if that cannot be done right away, then make contact by telephone.

WHY YOU SHOULD MEET WITH YOUR LAWYER RIGHT AWAY AND WHAT YOU SHOULD SEEK TO ACCOMPLISH

The Importance of a Litigation Strategy and Discovery Plan

To ensure that the meeting with your lawyer is as productive as possible, you should first read the complaint and try to discern from it what you are accused of having done or not done that supposedly makes you liable. If the complaint is what is known as a form complaint, this generally will be more difficult than if it is written by the plaintiff's counsel and sets forth some specific facts. However, in reading the complaint, you will at least be able to learn the identity of the plaintiff and when the event that allegedly resulted in injury occurred, even if it is a general form. Check your own records to see what they reveal about the plaintiff and to help refresh your memory. Make copies of these records so that you can review them without getting marks on your originals that could be misconstrued as attempts to alter the records. You will want to have reviewed whatever information you can quickly assemble before you meet with your attorney so that you can share all you recall about your role in treating the plaintiff. If there were others involved in the incident of treatment about which plaintiff complains, make some notes as to who they were, what role they played in that treatment, and how you know that they were involved or witnessed the treatment.

Ask your counsel for a facial evaluation of the complaint. What legal theories, other than negligence, is the plaintiff relying on? What are the necessary elements to those theories and how does your lawyer think the plaintiff will try to satisfy them? Are the theories asserted in the complaint's various causes of action supported in law? If not, should they be excised before trial by an appropriate motion?

Now, there are two things any good malpractice defense attorney will do to best represent a client: put together a *discovery plan* and a *litigation strategy.* The two go hand-in-hand, and although not all attorneys put them in writing, you will want a commitment from your attorney to do so for you. These are privileged documents, so your opponent will not be able to force you to disclose them. To be sure, both the initial discovery plan and litigation strategy will change as new information is learned and as there are rulings on motions filed by the parties that affect the course of the litigation. That is understandable, but it is important for you to have each revised plan because it will keep you informed as to how your defense is progressing, what needs to be done, by when, and whether the case is likely to be resolved without the necessity of trial. Your attorney will also likely work a little harder and maybe smarter for a client who shows interest in his or her own defense.

As already mentioned, your objective is to get rid of the case against you at the earliest opportunity, certainly before trial. Ask your attorney to explain his litigation strategy for accomplishing that goal. Is the complaint subject to a demurrer or motion to strike? If so, will these be filed or not; and if filed, when? Is the plaintiff asserting any claims that are outside the MICRA defenses available to you? Can those claims be disposed of by legal motions or are you stuck with defending hybrid claims? What evidence must be assembled to file a motion for summary judgment or summary adjudication? Does the discovery plan track with the litigation strategy so as to avoid time barriers that might otherwise preclude those motions from being filed?

Once you have a sense of the theories the plaintiff is relying on in suing you, it will be important to find out what evidence the plaintiff has, or must get, to tie you into each theory. Your attorney will develop a discovery plan that seeks to find out what you don't know and confirm what you do know. That discovery plan should set forth the facts essential to prove the elements of any theory of liability asserted and of any defense you will assert. Your attorney should seek a stipulation with opposing counsel as to material facts that you believe will not be disputed and put that stipulation in writing. The discovery plan should indicate the discovery device(s) that will be used to prove or disprove the existence of each element of all claims and defenses and the source of proof for each fact pertinent to those elements. The extent of claimed damages is something that you will want to nail the plaintiff down on.

What experts will your attorney need for your case? Will any of the treating physicians be treated as expert witnesses? How soon will these experts be retained? Do the local court rules limit the number of experts and, if so, does this hurt your defense? What experts has plaintiff's counsel used in the past for medical malpractice cases? (This information often can be ascertained through various computer database searches and by asking other counsel who may be familiar with or have litigated against the plaintiff's counsel in the past.)

CONCLUSION

John Wooden, the coach for UCLA's most successful winning basketball team, stated that "failing to prepare is preparing to fail." You and your defense team can best prepare to win by developing a well-thought-out and regularly revised plan for discovery and litigation strategy. In doing this, your sense of how the rules and players interact and can affect the outcome of the litigation game will make you a more valuable contributor in preparing to win.

3 Risk Reduction From a Plaintiff Attorney's Perspective

David Wm. Horan, MD, JD

SUMMARY

This chapter looks at malpractice litigation from the unique viewpoint of the plaintiff attorney. The necessary legal elements for a legally sound claim are discussed. What aspects of the doctor–patient relationship most affect the likelihood of litigation? What aspects of a physician's care, demeanor, and communication skills make him or her more or less formidable as a defendant? The chapter also discusses the physician's role in educating his or her own attorney and the preparation needed for a successful defense.

Key Words: Witness; negligence; communicating to a jury; risk reduction; working with your attorney; plaintiff's perspective.

INTRODUCTION

From a plaintiff attorney's perspective, risk reduction for a physician named in a malpractice claim is based on that physician's understanding of the way an experienced attorney approaches a potential medical negligence case. There is a widely held myth that a plaintiff attorney always uses professional witnesses who are paid to give expert testimony. That

From: *Medical Malpractice: A Physician's Sourcebook*
Edited by: R. E. Anderson © Humana Press Inc., Totowa, NJ

is untrue. The majority of plaintiff attorneys today use the best physician experts they can find to review a potential case. They are sent many cases and end up filing a very small percentage of them. To believe that the selected cases are built on the testimony of unreliable doctors is to give yourself a false sense of security and will increase the risk not only of being sued but also of being sued successfully.

This chapter is designed to give a basic understanding of the approach a plaintiff attorney uses in determining whether your case is the one that will be pursued. You first need to understand that keeping your patient away from an attorney's office is the first step; second, understand that if the patient gets to that office, then you need to know how to discourage the attorney from accepting the case and pursuing a claim against you.

BASIC UNDERSTANDING OF THE PROCESS

Just because a patient does not like the care he or she received or you personally does not mean he or she can sue you successfully. Although it is true that anyone can file a lawsuit, the time and money required to pursue litigation has made most plaintiff attorneys reluctant to accept a case that does not contain the three elements necessary to be successful in winning a lawsuit. These elements are negligence, proximate cause, and damage.

Negligence is defined as a deviation from the standard of medical care. *Standard of care* is defined as medical practice exercised with the same degree of skill used by physicians in your community under the same or similar circumstances. Demonstrating this is a very difficult burden to meet. It is only met by expert testimony.

Plaintiff attorneys know that juries will be persuaded only by the best possible expert medical witnesses. Do not deceive yourself by thinking that plaintiffs hire only paid "professional" experts. There may be isolated cases of this happening, but the majority of plaintiff attorneys know that even with the strongest case, juries want to believe the defendant doctor. Therefore, the plaintiff needs to get the best possible expert to overcome this innate bias in favor of the doctor.

Negligence means that you did something outside your area of expertise or did it in a fashion that others in your profession would not have done. This usually occurs when you try to do something new that you are not adequately trained for or when you do something in a careless way.

Risk reduction begins here. You can reduce your risk of a malpractice claim by documenting all possible complications in your records and explaining how and why they occurred. If you hide information, it will be found. Do not think that a plaintiff attorney will not find it. It is the explanation of an unexpected outcome that can reduce your risk of getting sued. If you have a complication, be forthcoming with the reason and explain to the patient why it occurred. If that patient enters an attorney's office, the lawyer can tell him that they are dealing with a complication rather than negligence. This scenario is played out every day in attorneys' offices. No attorney wants to put the time and money necessary to pursue litigation into a case involving an unavoidable complication. It is your chance to document your case in the record. Do not worry about this being a "red flag." If the patient is in the attorney's office, he already knows about the injury, and it is the cause that is the patient's concern.

Proximate cause is the link between the negligence and damages. The question is whether or not negligence directly caused the alleged injury. The damages must be shown to be real and, in most cases, permanent for there to be recovery sufficient to justify the time and money required to prepare the case and pursue litigation.

Remember that the plaintiff attorney usually has had the case referred by another lawyer who is not experienced in malpractice litigation. The plaintiff attorney is putting his or her own money into the case expenses, which he or she will get back only if the case is won. Thus, it is important for you to know that the early stages of review are done with utmost care to avoid accepting a case that has little chance of recovering damages. Your job is first to keep the patient out of the attorney's office. Then, if your patient does go to an attorney, you want your case to be the one that is turned down.

The knowledge that the plaintiff's attorney will only take a case involving probable negligence and not simply a mistake in judgment should guide your approach to an injured patient and the way you document complications or unexpected results in your records.

APPROACH TO PATIENTS

I am certain you have been told that your interpersonal relationship with the patient and his or her family is key to keeping the patient out of an attorney's office. I cannot emphasize this enough. From the plaintiff attorney's perspective, most patients simply want to know what happened when there was an unexpected result. Talk with the patient. Do not avoid the patient or hide the facts. In the majority of cases, an open and honest explanation will keep the patient from seeking answers from an attorney. Things can go wrong because medicine is not a precise science. It is a practice. It involves educating your patients. Just as a vaccine can help people avoid the flu, so, too, can good patient communication work in making patients feel that you are in this with them and are there to help if something goes wrong.

Do not feel that your openness will be held against you in a courtroom. Plaintiff attorneys are not going to win cases against doctors who are kind to their patients, try to help them, and take responsibility when an adverse outcome occurs. If you avoid discussing a complication with your patients, they will try to get answers either from other doctors, who may be critical of your care, or from an attorney. From a plaintiff attorney's perspective, nothing lowers your risk of being sued successfully as much as your documented frank explanation to the patient regarding what happened. That is what jurors feel distinguishes good doctors. The jury sees that something went wrong through no one's fault and that the doctor then worked hard to help the patient recover.

From an attorney's point of view, a doctor who has a complication but communicates openly and works to help his or her patient recover makes a very strong defendant. The jury will love that defendant doctor. However, plaintiff attorneys usually do not have to worry about this scenario because many doctors avoid discussing complications with their patients. This makes the physician appear guilty and they become a very weak defendant. Thus, my advice is to practice medicine with your patients' best interests in mind and treat them as you would like to be treated if you were the patient—especially when there is a complication. The patient gets an explanation and knows you care. That is the best form of risk management.

ONCE YOU ARE SUED,
WHAT SHOULD BE YOUR FIRST CONCERN?

If a claim is filed against you, the first thing you must be concerned about, after informing your insurance carrier, is the attorney who will defend you. You must feel comfortable with that individual in terms of his or her experience and interest in you. Do not worry if the attorney tells you he or she is busy; however, be certain that you feel he or she can focus on your case and provide you with the attention you will need.

You will need to educate your attorney about the case and to be honest with yourself about the quality of the care you have provided. Review a textbook and the recent literature on the subject matter; then give it to your attorney to review. You may need to educate him or her and it will pay off for you. You must understand that your efforts in educating your attorney about the medical aspects of the case will be worthwhile. You can be certain that the plaintiff attorney is doing the same research.

However, no one knows your case like you do. So put that knowledge to work. Make certain that the basic medical information that the plaintiff attorney certainly will have has been provided to your attorney.

From the plaintiff attorney's perspective, when doctors work closely with their attorneys, are not in denial about a lawsuit, and discharge their responsibilities to their patients, the chances of winning are diminished.

ONCE YOUR DEPOSITION IS SCHEDULED, THE PLAINTIFF ATTORNEY IS LOOKING FOR SPECIFIC THINGS

The order of the information the plaintiff attorney seeks is as important as their content. They are as follows:

1. How does the defendant physician react to people?
2. How does the defendant physician react to his or her attorney?
3. How does the defendant physician react to questions?
4. What is the expertise of the defendant physician?

If a jury likes you, it will be more likely to find for you. Thus, it is important for you to react to people in an accommodating manner. Do not be an arrogant, know-it-all doctor; many doctors appear to be. The effort you make in relating to those around you during the deposition and during the trial will be key to whether you are successful in the litigation.

You must respect and listen to your attorney. If you do not, the jury and the plaintiff lawyer will know it. Remember, law is not your area of expertise. If you do not respect your attorney, ask your insurance carrier for another one. Do not show your contempt or lack of respect for the justice system through your lack of respect for your attorney. Many doctors make this mistake.

Plaintiff attorneys are allowed to ask you questions during a deposition. If you are courteous and respectful when asked questions, the plaintiff attorney will conclude that you will behave that way in trial as well. To show respect and be the kind of caring doctor that jurors will love is not how a plaintiff attorney wants you to behave.

Study the medical aspects of the case and then teach them to your attorney. You may think you will remember the facts of the case simply by having experienced them, but you will be surprised at the details you have forgotten. However, you still must understand that this is the least important thing the plaintiff attorney is looking for when he or she assesses your ability to fight a potential suit. The most important thing is you and the impression you will make on a jury.

GENERAL CONCEPTS

Risk reduction from the plaintiff attorney's perspective really is very simple. If you are honest and straightforward with your patients when there is a complication and you are honest and straightforward to a jury, you have maximized your risk reduction. The attorney for the injured person must assess his or her ability to win in trial. That attorney is risking his or her time and money to pursue a case for which a fee will only be recovered if he or she wins. Attorneys assess you as they assess their chances.

The assessment takes place before the attorney ever meets you and is based on what you have written in your medical records. The attorney looks to see if you are honest and forthcoming, which is not something he or she wants to see in a potential defendant. Many doctors try to hide their mistakes from their patients. If you share your concerns with the patient when there is a complication, that openness will be a very effective deterrent to a plaintiff lawyer. You may feel you are raising a red flag by documenting that something is wrong. However, you may be keeping your patient from going to an attorney for answers, and you will be showing what a wonderful doctor (and witness) you will be if there is a lawsuit.

Your goal is to minimize the chances of your patient seeking legal aid to get answers. Your goal is also to be successful if all that occurred was a complication rather than a deviation from the standard of medical care. Hopefully, this chapter helps you understand some simple ways of accomplishing these goals.

4 The Physician As a Witness

Joel A. Mattison, MD, FACS

SUMMARY

This chapter is a personal reflection on the role of the physician as an expert witness in medical malpractice litigation. It looks at both the individual experience and professional obligations of the expert from both the medical and the legal perspectives. A number of practical suggestions for courtroom preparation and deportment are presented.

Key Words: Expert witness; courtroom strategy; courtroom deportment; cross-examination.

INTRODUCTION

When a physician has either the opportunity or the obligation to testify as an expert witness, the reaction often passes through a cascade of several phases.

- First, there is usually an overdose of humility: "Am I capable?" and "Can I learn enough about this matter to be of value in the courtroom?" *Humility is an asset, but it must be genuine and not an act.* Teddy Roosevelt once commented that the bravest man he had ever known was the one who followed him up San Juan Hill. Although this came from a hero, the arrogance of such a remark is apparent even, or especially, when subtle.

From: *Medical Malpractice: A Physician's Sourcebook*
Edited by: R. E. Anderson © Humana Press Inc., Totowa, NJ

- Will they take advantage of me? *They will certainly try. Be careful, but do not let your caution rob you of your effectiveness.*
- Can I avoid making an utter fool of myself? *It depends on how much of a head start you already have.*
- Why should I become involved? Is it a public responsibility or duty?
- Can I understand enough about courtroom behavior to be useful? *You must be willing to learn this carefully from the attorney who has engaged you.*
- Can I avoid impaling myself with my own imagined cleverness? *Yes, you can, so avoid all attempts at humor or fancy footwork.*
- Can I really help, at little or no risk to myself? *Everything in life has associated risks, and the courtroom is often a battleground. If this vulnerability frightens you, then think twice before you agree to testify or even to review a case.*
- Can I find any helpful information on how to be an effective expert? *Very little, because most effective experts tend to want to avoid sharing their strategies.* My wife's reaction to my writing this chapter was, "Are you going to give away all your trade secrets?" It is my hope that knowledge of a few principles will be of great assistance to those who are interested in facilitating the quest for justice. Moreover, not all of these strategies will be equally effective for everyone. Gather a lot of strategy but be careful not to try to use all of it in the same case.

SOME PRELIMINARY ADVICE

The following is a list of basic things to remember as you prepare for litigation in a malpractice suit.

1. Remember that although this may be your first time, it is a well-understood and familiar arena to those who are involved in it weekly or monthly. You are not likely to come up with any new or clever answers that have not already been heard by the judge, opposing counsel, and some of the jury. Remember to be always courteous and kind. This will take your adversaries by surprise and is a useful arrow in your quiver. If you cannot control your feelings and be objective, then this task is not for you.
2. The Apostle Paul advised to "be subject to those in authority." In the courtroom, this includes a descending hierarchy, at the bottom of which you will find yourself. Remember that the judge is deserving of the respect of his or her office and of his or her civil authority. Never try to be "funny" with the judge. It simply will not work, and

most judges under the pressure of their responsibilities will be somewhat short on humor. When you enter the courtroom, a nod to the
judge seems appropriate, but it should be carried no further. I usually
have made it a practice to do nothing until I am instructed (e.g., "Be
seated," etc.). I have rarely found it necessary to address the judge
during a trial, but I will occasionally pause and look toward him or
her to see if there is some forthcoming clarification to the question
just asked. This is a part of my personal philosophy that we should
assume nothing. Sometimes the judge may voluntarily clarify the
question or instruct you somewhat. If you are in too much of a hurry
and blurt out an answer, you may miss out on the only helpful advice
you may get on that day.

3. I have a brother-in-law who seems to be a very good businessperson.
   He has a single rule that he applies to all situations: "The first one to
   speak always loses." That has always been of great value in the courtroom and has often saved me from rushing down a rapid road to a
   wrong conclusion.

4. Always keep your temper under control. This is not optional. In fact,
   it is the very heart of the matter. Many cases are sabotaged through
   loss of personal control, even when the truth is on your side. This
   means never letting anyone get a rise out of you or cause you to return
   evil for evil. The jury, the adversaries, and the judge will lose respect
   for someone who lacks self-control—or who attempts to hold a higher
   opinion of him or herself than is justified.

5. When you do not understand a question perfectly, the response is
   simple: ask for clarification or an explanation. You should never
   answer a question that you do not fully understand. Sometimes you
   may have to apologize and ask again. If you still do not understand,
   you may use your own version of a response like:

   *"I am sorry, but I have to ask you for a little more help in
   understanding the question. It may not seem difficult, but I just
   cannot give an answer to fit what I understand you to have
   asked. Because I do not understand the question, I feel that I
   might risk giving an answer that is easily misunderstood, and
   even seem to lay aside my intent and oath to tell the truth, if I
   were to try to answer on the basis of the information that I seem
   to have been given."*

   Here, I will sometimes even ask the questioner for a pencil and paper
   to demonstrate my intention of getting to the answer (agreeing all the
   time that this seems to be an important question).

6. You must always be careful in citing textbooks, journals, and so on.
   It may be that on the next page you would have discovered some

statement that contradicts what you have interpreted previously. Be ready and be careful. The same goes for commenting about people. Some years ago, I was asked whether I knew Dr. John Marquis Converse (long-time professor of plastic surgery at New York University). Sensing some trap that was about to be sprung through the use of some obscure quote from Dr. Converse, I defused the situation by saying, "Yes, in fact I knew him back when he was still alive. Did you know that he married Gary Cooper's widow and that their daughter was the wife of Byron Janis, the concert pianist?" That line of questioning was quickly abandoned with a disappointed look.

7. If you are asked about whom you consider to be the outstanding expert on this matter, do not be afraid to imply or even to say that in this particular issue, in this patient, and under these circumstances, there is a constellation of facts and opinions, and that you are perhaps unique in having studied these relationships in preparing for this particular trial and have tried to put them into correct order accurately on the basis of your education, knowledge, and experience.

8. Be careful with your demeanor. When you cite your credentials, be careful not to sound as if you are boasting. Take on a spirit of humility and let your questioner discover the information that might otherwise appear to be a sign of arrogance if it came "voluntarily" from you, especially if your credentials are impeccable. I was once testifying in a fatal house fire case and pointed out the hot "zigger wire" spring scars in a projected photograph of the patient's thigh, a pattern providing proof that the patient had been burned in that same chair from which he was removed. This was a critical point in the trial. The plaintiff's attorney showed his irritation and replied, "I suppose that you are going to tell me that you are an expert on furniture, as well." I somewhat reluctantly provided the information that I was credentialed in furniture and household contents by two national appraisal organizations, had written articles on furniture, and had on more than one occasion spoken at Colonial Williamsburg on furniture of the 18th century although zigger wire was not used at that time. Without my having returned an angry comment to his opener, he dropped that line of questioning with a look of disgust (duly noted by the jury and even the judge).

9. This was the same trial about which the plaintiff's attorney had called me 1 hour before I was due to appear in court, telling me that I was excused and did not have to appear. I assured him that I did not trust this information and would be there, despite his advice. The first person I encountered on entering the courthouse was the trial judge, who knew nothing about my being excused. This was plainly

a clever trap, and it would likely have gotten me a citation for contempt of court.

10. Be very careful. I can recall once having set off a barrage of hostility from the questioning attorney and, wanting to make everyone positively aware of this, I apologized that I had embarrassed him unintentionally and publicly on his own ground and in front of his client, his colleagues, and even the judge. "Let's try to put that behind us and let me try again sincerely to answer your question."

11. It is difficult to cite or recommend a role model for the expert on the witness stand. I like to think that Andy Griffith, in his classic motion picture *No Time for Sergeants*, is very nearly the ideal, if not overdone. Although never obsequious, Griffith was simple (i.e., uncomplicated), pleasant, humble, always polite, and obliging in answering questions. He made every effort to be cooperative, and his pleasant and good-natured spirit always came through, never failing to irritate those who were trying to take advantage of him.

12. One must be careful not to appear either wise or a smart aleck on the stand. This will irritate everyone and will cave in on whomever attempts to use it.

13. Remember that the judge is always in charge in the courtroom. Any temporary victories by an expert witness will be short-lived under the withering stare of an experienced judge.

14. Also remember that the attorney who engaged your services is in charge of working out the strategy for the case presentation. The cleverest and best plan is of little use if it is brought up at the wrong time or out of sequence or if it is at cross-purposes with the strategy of the experienced attorney. You should discuss your ideas and suggestions with him or her and follow instructions.

15. The truth: Mark Twain once pointed out that no one has a sufficiently good memory to be a successful liar. Do not attempt to be the first. Always speak the truth as you understand it, and do not play with words in some clever attempt to disguise what you are saying. Longer-than-expected answers always invite the listeners to examine them with great care, and the tone and raised pitch of your voice will often reveal your anxiety. So also will giving more answer than the question justifies. Other signs of anxiety include dry mouth, stuttering, sputtering, repetition, and movement. Remember that we are always at our worst when anxiety has robbed us of whatever clear thinking and believability we may have brought to the task.

16. It is always good to look directly into the eyes of your questioner. Be in no hurry to answer. Smile occasionally, but make it a genuine smile and not a practiced one. With great care, you may occasionally

smile aside (impersonally) at some overzealous comment by an adversarial attorney. However, never argue, and never show your teeth.

17. When you have no idea of what your answer should be, you may use the strategy of looking directly at the questioner and saying, "I am so glad you asked that. I believe that this is a very important question with information that is important for the jury to have." (And then what is your answer?) Frequently, even the most experienced attorney will at least briefly wonder why he or she ever brought this point up, and it will thus often diffuse the strategy of a question that you believe to be irrelevant or misleading.

OTHER SOURCES

There are many helpful books for the beginning expert witness. One old standard was *The Art of Cross-Examination* by Francis L. Wellman. This book was originally copyrighted in 1903 and 1904 by The Macmillan Company, and later in 1933 and 1934 by Francis L. Wellman. Later still, the Dorset Press copyrighted it in 1986. It is of great benefit to read some classic courtroom questions and answers, but only for purposes of illustration and not for your own use. However, be aware of the consequences of trying to be innovative in someone else's field.

OTHER ADVICE

Your relationship with the attorney with whom you are working is extremely important. Believe and trust him or her by giving him or her all your relevant theories so that he or she can decide whether and how to use them. I cannot remember ever having gone to trial without my attorney having questioned me at length. It is especially helpful when someone actually seats you at the witness stand during the lunch hour and browbeats you so that you will have experienced trial by fire. No one has ever refused to do this when I requested it, and the browbeating session was always more severe than the actual event. This is not a rehearsal for effective testimony; rather, it is a means of seeing whether or how well you can hold everything together under duress, allowing you to become familiar with the possible worst-case scenario presented by opposing counsel.

On one occasion, a doctor joke was tried out on me when I was on the stand. Very calmly and sadly, I said that I had been taught even as a child never to make light of someone else's profession. (It was an old joke anyway and not really humorous.) The questioner soon regretted his attempt to embarrass me. Although he was late in recognizing it, he lost his professional decorum and spent some time recovering it.

You are sworn to tell the truth. Do not forget that, and make no exceptions. If an answer seems as if it might be detrimental, do not play around with words and try to disguise the truth so that you think it might be more helpful. Your change in demeanor and the pitch of your voice will give you away. Be direct and answer truthfully. A long and convoluted answer will always raise suspicions, especially with an attorney who understands this and will attempt to use it.

A word about dress and grooming: Do not pick your best or worst suit, but if you do not have a suit, go out and buy a conservative model, and make certain that it fits. Make it dark or at least a sincere blue. To me, a neutral shirt or blouse is a white one. No one will give you extra credit for the latest style. Avoid any jewelry that calls attention to itself. An old rule is that you should look at yourself in a full-length mirror and remove whatever first captures your attention. Do not get in your own way.

When you are seated, the attorney will usually look at you and smile disarmingly. He or she may even greet you, and that greeting should be acknowledged with a return and a smile. During the time you are on the stand, you must be relaxed and unthreatened, pleasantly keeping your guard up.

The questions will usually progress from fairly simple to very complex. Expect this. Usually, a seeming easing of the questions will gradually diffuse your attention and caution. Watch out! One of England's best known executioners would frequently show up early enough to hide his "sword of justice" beneath the straw around the block at center stage. He would then speak comfortingly to his subject and suddenly without any warning the act was done. We may not like how he earned his living, but everyone saw him as compassionate, even under the worst and most ghastly circumstances.

As with everyone else, some attorneys are openly hostile, whereas others may seem friendly, seeking to gain your confidence. At this point, you may even think, "I believe that this fellow likes me." This is a dangerous moment. At such a time when you have been disarmed, questions can slip by you without your being aware of even the direction from which the darts are coming (or have just gone). Never drop your guard. The next thing you feel will likely be the tightening of the noose. Be careful and always avoid the look of surprise.

You are supposed to look and to behave like some sort of a Marcus Welby to everyone. Be loveable and kind beyond any doubt. For you to do your best job, the jury must see you as warm, friendly, and eager to cooperate. More than that, they must like you. Always be yourself, but try to hold your answers in your mouth just long enough to run them through twice, as you think of what you are saying and how it may sound. Kindness is the thought and the word for the day.

Avoid looking at your watch. Your most important task for today is to tell the truth, and you do not want to appear to be in a rush to do so. It never hurts to have an extra copy of your curriculum vitae with you, but do not offer it unless asked.

I always feel that answers should be short, especially when not directly related to the matter at hand. If the answer is too short, you will be asked again. Be careful not to give more information than requested.

When you recognize a question as one that has already been asked, politely ask if the questioner remembers having already asked that question, and comment emotionlessly that you thought you had given a satisfactory answer.

Remember the Boy Scout motto: "Trustworthy, loyal, helpful, friendly, courteous, obedient, cheerful, thrifty, kind, brave, clean, and reverent." You should be careful to review these from time to time and seek to exemplify them, in or out of court.

Be careful how you express yourself. Any double entendre, hint of disrespect, demeaning intent, vulgarity, or even mild profanity can destroy your image. George Washington said that profanity was the result of an inability to express oneself otherwise.

There is little use in trying to learn anything about the courtroom from television or Perry Mason movies. These are for entertainment and often at the expense of the truth. However, you can study films and videos for the various ways in which exaggerated surprise is registered by a witness, an attorney, or the defendant. The sudden increased separation of the eyelids, dropping of the jaw, or motion of the hands are all instant conditioned responses that everyone in the courtroom can recognize. Be especially careful not to laugh inappropriately or at an inopportune moment. If your hands seem shaky or tremulous, put them beneath the top of the witness box desk. Do not announce your uneasiness publicly.

If attacked personally, imperceptibly bow your head and give thanks, because here is your real opportunity to gain the sympathy of the jury. You may look hurt but never angry. The worse the attack, the greater your opportunity to turn this to your advantage. No one likes to see someone attacked, especially if unfairly, and this is the supreme opportunity for you to turn the tide of sympathy in your favor.

BE READY

Listen to the question! Remember the old saw, "Can you state your name, please?" The answer to this question is, "Yes." These words must never be used in court, but they will serve to remind you to tell the truth and not to volunteer any information, even if you feel it might be helpful.

You will probably be asked how much you are billing for your courtroom appearance. Be careful not to invite even more attention by attempting to dodge the issue. A good answer is usually, "I am not charging any fee for my appearance and testimony. I am simply billing for the time I have to absent myself from the duties of my practice to review this matter carefully and to be here today." (This seems disingenuous at best and contradicts the next sentence.) I prefer to give a figure of my charges in terms of per hour rather than in a lump sum (of which I can hardly be aware until the matter is concluded).

Be able to estimate what percent of your income is derived from your work as an expert witness, as distinguished from your professional income.

You also may subtly point out that you believe that your study and opinion of the case may make it an easier matter to deliberate and that you see this as a citizen's duty.

Be prepared to answer whether you sometimes testify for the plaintiff and at others for the defense. Many people feel that this credits you with objectivity. I will sometimes explain that I try to represent the truth in such a way that it stands on its own and is not for or against either party. Many times, I have testified at trial concerning motor vehicular accidents (and others) by whichever side needs and asks for me.

When asked what you have read or studied in preparation for this trial, have a list of all depositions you have reviewed, a list of journals that you regularly read, and anything else that is out of the ordinary. Frequently, I am asked what publications I "subscribe to." My reply is that my occupation as a medical director in a large hospital allows me the privilege of using the hospital's medical library, where I usually spend parts of 3 days every week reading and searching for information that will be important for me to print as editor of our hospital's monthly physician newsletter. This is aside from the time spent in meetings, continuing medical education, conferences, and rounds. I am especially aware of the importance of knowledge of the history of medicine. I am also managing editor of the *Journal of the American Board of Quality Assurance and Utilization Review Physicians.*

WHY IS THE EXPERT WITNESS
NECESSARY IN COURT?

The answers to this question are as follow:

- Medicine, like law, is a very esoteric discipline, and the various legal experts may not be able (without assistance from other disciplines) to rank matters according to meaningful, objective, and just priorities.

- Under most circumstances, justice may be served by an additional slant or other viewpoint that may tend to be more objective, if the witness seems inclined to take such a viewpoint.

- There will be questions and issues that need third-party clarification.

- The expert is not there to "get anyone off" but is in the role of "teacher," which is one of the basic duties of a physician. As such, he or she should be able to clarify many issues that are not immediately clear.

- The expert is expected to have "been there" in previous cases based on similar principles to bring the point of view of experience in addition to knowledge.

- the expert helps keep matters relevant and in balance so that one side is not able to easily intimidate or to distort.

- To put the expert in the crucible just long enough to examine his or her prejudices or lack of objectivity. This keeps most of us honest and helps to facilitate the quest for truth and justice.

We are all aware that imperfections and misunderstandings may distort the pure intent of seeking justice, and sadly, we have to note that some experts are easily swayed by prejudice in favor of the client of the lawyer who engaged them. This can often be ameliorated by the opposing attorney, or the opposing expert, so that at least both viewpoints are clearly present at trial. The right of decision making belongs to the jury alone and not to the expert.

The expert witness need not be intimidated by his or her lack of knowledge of the law. The expert is present to serve the needs of both attorney and the jury. The expert who sees him or herself as a "gladiator" or a "gun for hire" will not usually be effective in the pursuit of justice, although he or she may well be able to sway a jury. It should not about "my people" (i.e., experts) being better than "your people," even though the side with the best and clearest experts has a definite advantage.

Probably the last and least desirable quality of an expert witness is the irrepressible desire to win at all costs and by whatever distortion is necessary. This is not an ego trip. If this appears to be the case, then the expert's testimony will be severely and deservedly discounted.

What ethic serves to guide the expert witness? Very simply, it is the ninth commandment: "Thou shalt not bear false witness against thy neighbor." This is a simple admonition that requires no commentary. The oath to tell the truth is serious and binding. You should leave the witness stand with everyone's respect, including and especially your own.

5 The Judicial Process

Discovery and Deposition

Jonathan I. Epstein, MD

SUMMARY

This chapter explores the nature and conduct of pretrial discovery and the deposition process from the physician's point of view. Practical suggestions for witness preparation and guides to recognition of the methods, procedures, and goals of the plaintiff attorney are presented. Courtroom deportment is discussed, and model questions and appropriate responses are included.

Key Words: Deposition; interrogatory; discovery; medical malpractice.

INTRODUCTION

There are several aspects to the process of discovery. The first aspect is production requests. During this phase, documents, slides, and X-rays may be requested. During written interrogatories, the plaintiff attorney will pose a limited number of detailed written questions for you (in conjunction with your attorney) to reply to under oath *(1,2)*. Another aspect to discovery is oral interrogation, also known as a *deposition*. Well before the deposition, the defendant should insist on a meeting with his or her lawyer. This will allow time to know what is expected of you. Also, if something new or unexpected arises, there will be time to deal with it. It is reasonable to have someone from your

From: *Medical Malpractice: A Physician's Sourcebook*
Edited by: R. E. Anderson © Humana Press Inc., Totowa, NJ

attorney's office cross-examine you as part of your preparation. It is important to note that everything you write is discoverable except for direct communications to your lawyer. Consequently, if you are going to keep written notes, it is advised that you record only facts and not opinions.

DISCOVERY: DEPOSITION

The purpose of a deposition is discovery by both sides so that there are no surprises at trial. The deposition is the most important event for the defendant physician before trial *(1–7)*. The location of the deposition may vary. It is often held in the plaintiff attorney's office. However, one can ask to have it in a setting in which the pathologist feels more comfortable, such as in the hospital. The deposition is typically attended by a court reporter, who will record everything. Also present will be your attorney and the plaintiff attorney. There may be other defense attorneys present if they represent other parties within the lawsuit, such as codefendant physicians or the hospital. The possibility exists that the plaintiff's family could also be present. The deposition is taken under oath and can be read to the jury at trial. The format of the deposition is for the opposing (plaintiff's) attorney to pose a series of questions (cross-examination). Your defense attorney will follow, typically with fewer questions, to clarify certain points raised during cross-examination. Bring your curriculum vitae, but do not bring literature or notes because they will be discoverable.

There are several underlying purposes of the deposition. These are described here.

Plaintiff's Goal: To Be Educated
About Your Strategies and Information

The defendant's or physician's role is not to educate the opposing attorneys, but rather just to answer their questions:

- Do not volunteer unnecessary information. If you provide them with information they did not request, it may deprive your attorney of determining when certain information will be disclosed for maximal impact.
- In general, answer questions with either a simple yes or no or short, complete sentences. Providing a lengthy discourse may open up further questions or opinions that may be detrimental to your case.
- A common ploy will be for the plaintiff's lawyers to pause for long periods of time. Do not feel the need to fill in the silence. The attorney

may be waiting for you to offer additional information that could eventually be damaging to your case.

- Do not agree to supply any information or documents to the plaintiff attorney. Rather, these requests should be made to your lawyer.

Plaintiff's Goal: To Impeach Your Credibility

What you answer at deposition is sworn testimony and can be read back at trial to make you look bad if there are certain internal inconsistencies or differences in trial testimony. The role of the physician in this regard is to tell the truth and to be consistent.

- Even if there is a relatively inconsequential fact, always be truthful. Assume that any misstatement will be discovered, and it will be made to look like nothing that you say can be trusted.
- If you do not know something or are unsure about an answer, respond by saying, "I don't know," or, "I don't remember." You will not appear stupid; rather, you will not get yourself into trouble by saying something that may be incorrect. Do not make statements such as, "Honestly, I don't remember." This implies that otherwise you are not honest.
- Avoid statements such as, "I always," or, "I never," because these typically are not true.
- Always pause before answering a question. This allows you to think carefully before answering, and it allows time for your attorney to raise objections.
- Always try to be consistent with answers that you have already given.
- If you make a mistake, acknowledge it and clarify your prior responses. Do not panic, because these mistakes can be rehabilitated at trial or when your attorney follows up with questions.
- If you remember something or have a new insight, wait until a recess and first discuss it with your counsel in private.

The following are some specific ploys used by plaintiff lawyers to ruin your credibility.

Plaintiff attorney:

Asks specifically ambiguous questions so that you will answer them in an incriminating manner.

Defending physician:

Do not help the plaintiff attorney by saying, "Do you mean X or Y?" The plaintiff attorney may not even know about X or Y, and now that you have educated him or her, he or she will ask you about each of these issues, potentially hurting your case. If you do not hear the question, respond, "Please repeat the question." If you do not understand a question, respond, "Please clarify the question." However, do not overdo it.

Requesting that questions be repeated multiple times may make you look somewhat stupid.

Plaintiff attorney:
Asks compound questions.

Defending physician:
Respond by saying, "There are two points raised by your question, and let me answer each one of them separately."

Plaintiff attorney:
Uses double-negatives in an attempt to confuse the physician.

Defending physician:
Ask for the statement to be clarified without the use of double negatives or carefully try to dissect the question and answer it correctly.

Plaintiff attorney:
Uses hypothetical questions. Often, a hypothetical question will include facts different than you believe to be true for your case. If you just answer the question, then it can be used out of context at trial in a damaging fashion.

Defending physician:
Answer a hypothetical question in this way: "Although this hypothetical question does not apply to the current case, if I assume the facts in your hypothetical question, then I would answer as follows." In this way, the entire sentence when it is read at trial will not be misleading.

Plaintiff attorney:
Asks if some text or individual is authoritative. Asks what textbooks to which you commonly refer or recommend, so that if something is found within that text that conflicts with your testimony, you can be made to look bad.

Defending physician:
The answer is, "Nothing is authoritative." Authoritative means that 100% of what is written or 100% of what a person says is the truth. The correct way to respond to this question is, "Nothing in its entirety is authoritative, but I would have to see specifically the sentence or section on a specific issue to see if I agree with that statement." Respond to the question on what text you recommend by saying, "I rely on my training, experience, multiple books, and the literature in general."

Plaintiff attorney:
Summarizes your testimony, yet twists it to support his or her case.

Defending physician:
Watch out for phrases such as, "Is it fair to say," or, "Do you mean to say this?" The best way to respond to these questions is to say, "That

is not what I said," and then go forward and repeat your testimony in your own words. Specifically clarify any inaccuracies that he or she made in his or her summary.

Plaintiff attorney:
Asks you about someone else's motivation.

Defending physician:
Never speculate. One cannot know what is in someone else's mind. Do not use answers such as, "I think," or, "In my opinion." Only state specific facts.

Plaintiff attorney:
Quotes from a record or a document and asks you questions.

Defending physician:
To not misspeak, always ask to read the document before commenting on it.

Plaintiff attorney:
Asks questions that could be misleading if you answer them with a simple yes or no. For example, assume a case of prostatic atrophy misdiagnosed as adenocarcinoma. The attorney may ask, "When due skill and care are used by a pathologist, can he usually distinguish between atrophy and cancer?"

Defending physician:
If you merely answer in the affirmative, it implies negligence. Rather, you should expand your answer by stating, "Although you can usually distinguish between the two processes, there are cases when it can be very difficult to tell them apart."

Plaintiff attorney:
Asks if something is true all of the time.

Defending physician:
Nothing in medicine is true 100% of the time. All you can say is what is more probable than not, which is also known as a reasonable degree of medical certainty (>50%).

Plaintiff attorney:
Asks, "Are you sure that is all you have to say on the subject?" If you say yes and later more information surfaces, then it looks like you were trying to withhold information.

Defending physician:
Respond, "That is all that I can think of at the present time."

Plaintiff attorney:
Interrupts you in mid-sentence, making what you say a half-truth.

Defending physician:
Let the plaintiff attorney finish, and then state firmly and courteously that you were interrupted and that you had not finished your answer. Either he will let you finish your answer, or your lawyer will be able to ask you the question after the plaintiff attorney is finished.

Plaintiff's Goal:
To Judge How Effective a Witness You Will Be at Trial

How you do at deposition will be factored in as to whether the case may be settled or not. The following are some guidelines for you to consider.

- You should come across as knowledgable, polite, calm, and professional and show that you care for the patient.
- It is critical for you to control your emotions and not show arrogance. Lawyers can make outrageous claims against physicians in malpractice cases. As long as they make it in the setting of a court or deposition, they are immune against claims of defamation.
- Dress professionally.
- Never use even the mildest obscenity.
- There is no such thing as "off the record." If a plaintiff attorney hears you say something during a break, he or she can ask you about it on the record.
- Do not joke. This can be made to imply that you are not taking the case seriously.

TYPES OF PLAINTIFF ATTORNEYS AT DEPOSITION

One author has aptly described plaintiff attorneys as "pals," "freight trains," "butterflies," "time bombs," or "ignoramuses"(8).

Pal

A deposition can appear informal. In part, this may relate to the setting. Also, attorneys may be casually dressed, joking with each other, often including your lawyer in this banter before the deposition starts. Remember that the deposition is adversarial and that their role is to make you look bad. Do not let the "pal" plaintiff attorney disarm you with his or her friendliness.

Freight Train

The "freight train" plaintiff attorney will barrel along with rapid-fire questions, trying to make you speak before you think. The best way to handle this type of attorney is to hesitate before answering each question and to respond in complete sentences, which will slow down the process and ruin the timing of the plaintiff attorney.

Butterfly

The "butterfly" plaintiff attorney flips from one line of questioning to another in an attempt to confuse you. The goal of the plaintiff attorney is to make you give conflicting testimony. He or she will ask the same question in multiple ways over different points of time in the deposition, hoping for inconsistent answers. The key is to be consistent and to think before you answer. Do not worry about the apparent confusion in terms of the line of questioning. Concentrate on the questions at hand, and answer in a consistent manner.

Time Bomb

The "time bomb" plaintiff attorney saves the most difficult questions for the end of the deposition when you are most tired. You can ask for a break if you are tired or if you need to use the restroom. During the break, you can discuss the situation with your lawyer. Just make sure that this discussion is out of earshot of the plaintiff attorney.

Ignoramus

The apparently ignorant plaintiff attorney tries to get you to volunteer information that you otherwise would not. Assume the opposing attorney is well-versed in the subject and do not overly educate him or her.

OBJECTIONS RAISED DURING DEPOSITION

Your attorney can object for many different reasons. Some of these include if the plaintiff attorney has already asked you the same question multiple times. Your attorney may object, "asked and answered." Other common objections include those to leading, ambiguous, and all-inclusive questions.

When your attorney objects, take a second to think about why the objection is occurring. However, do not be overly concerned about the objections so that you lose your concentration. Most objections are nothing to worry about and are procedural. After an objection has been raised, you can still answer the question if your attorney says so. Later, the judge may make a ruling to strike a question.

POSTDEPOSITION

You will be offered the opportunity to read your deposition and to correct any errors in how the transcriber heard you. If you want to make substantial changes, then ask your attorney. In general, any changes made to the deposition that are substantial will look damaging. Some jurisdictions will allow such substantial changes to the deposition and others will not. Read a deposition carefully. If there are any discrepancies in what you said in the deposition, as opposed to what you will say at trial, then prepare how to explain them. You should have a postdeposition meeting to assess the case and your ability to defend it successfully. You should also ask your attorney about reading other depositions in the case. For example, reading the plaintiff's deposition will show how he or she sees the case and what arguments may be used during the case. It is debatable whether you should sit in on other depositions. The potential advantage of sitting in on some depositions is that the plaintiff's expert and plaintiff may be more truthful in the presence of the defending physician. The disadvantage is that depositions take time away from your practice, and it is hard to listen to an expert impugning you. If you do sit in on a deposition and something is said on which you want to comment to your lawyer, make a note of it and discuss it with him or her in private. Before your trial, read your deposition carefully, and virtually memorize it so that you will be consistent at trial.

Before your court date, visit the courtroom to familiarize yourself with the setting. Plan on attending the entire trial, demonstrating that you care about the case. You will be sitting next to your attorney throughout the trial. It is also reasonable to have your spouse attend the trial once or twice to show your human side. When sitting in the courtroom and during other testimony, make eye contact with the jury. Identify inaccuracies made by other witnesses or points that can be used by your attorney, which can be discussed with your attorney when there is a break in the case. The following are some guidelines on handling yourself at trial (*see* the Discovery: Deposition section for how to answer questions posed by the plaintiff attorney)(*1–3,8–10*).

1. When it is time for your testimony, dress conservatively. Men are encouraged to wear dark suits, and subtle ties, but not bow ties, which have an eccentric connotation. Individuals should not wear tinted glasses. Heavy jewelry, fancy jewelry, and expensive watches should not be worn.

2. Sit straight in the witness chair without fidgeting.

3. Face halfway between the jury and lawyer. Turn to face the lawyer when he or she poses a question and then turn to the jury to answer the question.

4. Be sincere and be yourself. The jury expects some minor degree of nervousness. Do not try to come across cocky and arrogant. Show that you care and be human.

5. Keep answers short and simple. People tend to tune out during lengthy explanations.

6. Do not use medical terminology that the jury will not understand, but also try not to talk down to the jury. The use of models, diagrams, and photographs can help illustrate points clearly.

7. Anticipate a hard time at trial. The plaintiff attorney will try to challenge your reputation and make you nervous. Jurors expect attorneys to be arrogant and aggressive, in part based on portrayals of attorneys by the media. On the other hand, jurors expect the physician to always be composed. No matter what, control your emotions as much as you can. Answer questions calmly and directly, even if under fire. Never become argumentative. Recognize that the plaintiff attorney is just doing his or her job. He or she has nothing personal against you. I have been involved in several cases in which the same attorney who grilled me on one case asked if he could hire me on a different case because I did such a good job under fire at a deposition. If you recognize that these attorneys are only doing what is expected of them, it may help in removing some of the emotion from the situation.

8. Do not look to your attorney for help during trial. This undermines your credibility and the appearance of independence.

9. Outside the courtroom, either before, during, or after breaks, always retain your professional demeanor. Do not joke, giggle, and so forth. Jurors could see you and think that you are not taking the case seriously. Also, do not talk about the case until your lawyers says it is okay, because the other side can pick up remarks.

ACKNOWLEDGMENT

This is an excerpt from an article entitled "Pathologists and the Judicial Process: How to Avoid It" by Jonathan I. Epstein, MD (Am J Surg Pathol 2001;25(4):527–537). It is reprinted with permission. This portion of the article was selected because it explains so well the purpose of pretrial discovery and provides valuable insight into the conduct of a deposition.

REFERENCES

1. Dodd MM, Dodd MJ. Anatomy of a medical malpractice lawsuit. Md Med J 1996;45:108–115.

2. Bounds JA. Introduction to notification, deposition, and court testimony. Neurol Clin 1999;17:335–343.
3. Finger AL. How to be your own best expert witness. Med Economics 1999;76: 96–100.
4. Horsley JE. Don't let your deposition be used against you. Med Economics 1995; 72:220–230.
5. Martello J. The deposition. The defendant's perspective. Clin Plast Surg 1999;26: 87–90.
6. Martin K, Cepero K. Discover strategies for avoiding legal pitfalls if you must ever give a deposition. Nursing 1999;29:60,61.
7. Metzger JP. Preparing for a deposition. Med Malpract Law Strat 1991;8:5–7.
8. Marshall JC. Credibility: the key to the successful physician witness. Surv Ophthalmol 1995;40:69–72.
9. Martello J. Trials, settlements, and arbitration. Clin Plast Surg 1999;26:97–101.
10. Martello J. Basic medical legal principles. Clin Plast Surg 1999;26:9–14.

III THE CLINICAL FACE OF LITIGATION

6 Communication and Patient Safety

Mark Gorney, MD

SUMMARY

Faulty communication is among the most common underlying causes of medical error and frequently erodes the doctor–patient relationship. Communication should be understood in the broadest sense, including nonverbal, oral, and written. This chapter reviews the most common mechanisms responsible for communication failures and recommends specific routines to minimize or avoid them altogether.

Key Words: Poor listening habits; nonverbal; speech tempo; body language; repetition.

INTRODUCTION

Patient anger underlies many malpractice claims and frequently results from ineffective communication. The breakdown is usually between doctor and patient but may also involve miscommunication between physicians and nurses or between physicians and family members.

Mastering the art of listening and increasing one's awareness of both verbal and nonverbal expression are important aspects of contemporary medical practice. Patients are increasingly assuming responsi-

From: *Medical Malpractice: A Physician's Sourcebook*
Edited by: R. E. Anderson © Humana Press Inc., Totowa, NJ

bility for their health care and often come to the doctor armed with information they have obtained from health-related websites on the Internet. They expect the doctor to listen to their complaints. They often have sufficient knowledge about their condition to ask intelligent questions, which may make the physician defensive, evasive, or hostile. This may be perceived by the patient as arrogance, leading to feelings of frustration, disappointment, and anger.

LISTENING

Hearing and listening are dissimilar processes. Listening is an active, cognitive process that involves interpreting what is heard and deciding on a response.

Most of our waking day is spent in some form of communication, and much of that time is listening. In the office and at the bedside, the amount of time a physician spends listening is even greater. According to Edward Kelsay (1), of the four basic communication skills (listening, speaking, reading, and writing), listening is the least apt to be formally taught.

Dr. Ralph G. Nichols of the University of Minnesota, a nationally recognized authority and researcher on the nuances of listening, believes that effective listening requires conscious effort (2). Busy physicians are at high risk of falling into poor listening behaviors. Nichols has identified the following 10 bad habits in listening behaviors that can lead to serious doctor–patient misunderstandings.

1. Dismissing the subject matter as uninteresting. A subconscious resistance to listening may arise if we become bored while listening to complaints that we have heard many times before from many other patients. Effective listening requires attention, patience, and, above all, suppression of the urge to control the conversation or "move it along."

2. Feigning attention. We all learn to look attentive during dull and boring meetings or to appear engaged during conversations that do not interest us. However, feigning attention is risky when talking with patients because they often sense when the doctor is merely pretending to listen and are apt to feel insulted.

3. Losing interest in verbose explanations. The media incessantly bombards us with professionally prepared "sound bites" and "happy talk." This may dull our ability to listen to a patient's often lengthy and unfocused explanations of symptoms that demand more of our active thought processes and time.

4. Allowing distractions. The physician's office environment is characterized by continuous interruptions (e.g., phone, intercom, and fax) that

disrupt physician–patient communications. Try to minimize office distractions that interrupt your attention when conversing with a patient.

5. Becoming distracted by the speaker. Instead of listening to what the patient says, one can easily become distracted by the patient's mannerisms or physical characteristics. This interferes with focusing on what the patient is saying.

6. Listening only for facts. Medical training and patient care is oriented toward objective observations and quantitative data. Doctors often fail to take into account the equally important emotional overtones and behavior of the patient as reflected in their comments and conversation.

7. Becoming distracted by the presentation. If you become enamored by a person's speaking style or manner of presentation, you are likely to suspend judgment about what the speaker is actually saying.

8. Allowing emotion-laden words that arouse antagonism. Certain words or phrases can trigger negative emotional reactions in the listener. For example, if you exert extraordinary effort on a patient's behalf and are then told, "You were just too busy for me," you are likely to feel antagonistic toward that person.

9. Note-taking. Although note-taking is essential to documenting a patient's history, it can distract your concentration or continuity of thought and increase the patient's anxiety. It is best to listen and make eye contact with the patient until a clear message is detected. It is best to jot down only important key words or phrases that help you reconstruct the conversation later.

10. Wasting the advantage of thought–speech speed. Most people speak at approx 125 words per minute but are capable of assimilating approx 500 spoken words per minute. The extra time is often used to think about something other than what the speaker is saying. Communication is more effective if you focus only on what is being said.

Listening Skills

Patients often base their assessment of a physician's competence more on communication skills than clinical talent. Some doctors have the ability to make each patient feel that whatever the patient is saying is the most important thing he or she has heard all day. Other physicians who may be just as qualified may appear impatient or uninterested. Experts on effective communication agree on the following simple rules for avoiding misinterpretation.

1. Reflective feedback. This technique informs the speaker whether or not his or her message is being heard and understood. This is accomplished by asking questions, making statements, or offering visual cues that indicate your understanding and degree of concurrence.

2. Silence. By remaining silent when a patient is speaking, you are less likely to be preparing or rehearsing your response while listening. Instead, focus on what is being said.
3. Positioning. Your own body language is a powerful communicator of attentiveness. For example, a too-relaxed posture can reflect disinterest, whereas arms crossed in front of your body often signals defensiveness. Some doctors avoid sitting behind a desk to remove a semblance of a barrier. If you lean forward slightly and look at the patient while he or she speaks, your nonverbal communication says, "I'm interested in what you have to say. Please continue" *(3,4)*.

SPEAKING: VERBAL AND NONVERBAL EXPRESSION

After listening to the patient, you need to respond. The following techniques help improve communication.

Tempo of Speech and Tone of Voice

Some physicians have a tendency to speak rapidly or to economize on words. To ensure that patients understand you, speak slowly and clearly. Often, the stress that physicians experience in their daily practice is reflected unconsciously in their tone of voice. For example, the phrase, "You should have called me," can be said in an empathic, solicitous manner or in an impatient, accusatory way. The effect that these two styles have on a patient can differ dramatically.

Pause for Assimilation and Feedback

When your message is complex, pause frequently, even if you do not sense confusion in the listener. A break in speech allows patients to either digest what you are saying or ask for clarification. In addition, repeatedly invite questions. The resulting dialogue reinforces the patients' feeling that they are participating in their health care. There is nothing wrong with asking, "Do you understand?" as often as you deem necessary. Most patients will interpret this question for what it is—a sincere interest in their welfare.

One of the best ways to ensure that explanations or instructions are understood is to ask patients to repeat what they have just been told. Explaining that you want to ensure their well-being can dispel the notion that you are being condescending. You might want to give the example that "50" and "15" sound very similar, but the numbers can literally spell the difference between life and death when they represent milligrams prescribed for a potent drug.

TAILOR YOUR LANGUAGE

One of the most common complaints in patient attitude surveys has to do with physicians' use of complex terminology or medical jargon. There is a substantial choice of words available for communicating with patients according to their intellectual and educational level. The goal is to make sure you are understood.

Whereas physicians define the stomach as a specific organ, patients complaining of a "stomach ache" might be referring to an indefinite area from the ribs to the pubis.

When you describe a procedure, choose words that do not produce anxiety. For example, "excise" might be misunderstood, whereas "cutting it out" sounds painful. "Removing it" is a better way to convey the message without inducing stress.

Repetition

Various studies have shown that the average patient retains only 35% of what he or she is told. To improve retention, summarize the essential points of your message at the end of the consultation or examination.

Request Written Questions

A visit to the doctor can cause anxiety that makes patients forget important questions or information until they have left the office. Encourage patients to write down questions and to bring a list on their next visit. If your patient already has a list, then do not, by word or body language, express impatience about answering the questions. In the event of an unfavorable outcome, the time you spent answering questions may avert a malpractice claim.

Body Language

Body language is as important when speaking as when listening. Starting with the first friendly handshake, nonverbal communication is important for establishing and maintaining patient confidence. Body language becomes absolutely critical if things start to go wrong. In speaking, as in listening, eye contact is critical and holds the patient's attention. A patient's facial expressions and frequent nods indicate how effectively you are getting your message across.

Do not permit your own emotions or frustrations to affect the patient. The anxieties of sick or injured people often act as a lens that greatly magnifies the physician's body language. A frown or a simple "hmmmm" by you may exacerbate that anxiety. In some cases, an innocent sigh, a raised eyebrow, or a look of skepticism when evaluating a colleague's results has triggered a patient's visit to an attorney.

Likewise, remember that a reassuring smile, a comforting touch, and a confident and caring attitude are indispensable ingredients for the development of solid doctor–patient relationships. Positive rapport can weather many treatment failures and complications.

PROBLEMS OF NURSE–PHYSICIAN COMMUNICATION

Case 1

A 39-year-old man was brought to the emergency room (ER) of a large hospital shortly after being struck in the head with a baseball bat. He was adequately evaluated and then discharged. Eleven days later, he returned to the ER because of increasing lethargy. He was hospitalized, and a computed tomography (CT) scan raised the question of a subdural hematoma. It was late in the evening when the CT scan was interpreted, and the patient was alert, so his physician decided to wait until morning to perform further studies.

When the patient's doctor left the hospital at 10 PM, he wrote orders for the nurses to check the patient's vital signs hourly. However, the doctor did not give specific direction to note the state of the patient's pupils or his state of consciousness or to call the doctor if any alteration occurred. He later said he felt it was unnecessary to leave such detailed directions because the nurses should have understood their duty in this regard.

However, the nurses were not alert to a progressive deterioration that occurred during the night. It was not until the patient was comatose at 4 AM that a neurosurgeon was called. A craniotomy at 6 AM identified a subdural hematoma. Death occurred 5 days later.

At trial, several negligence issues arose, but the plaintiff's attorney mainly concentrated on failed communications—failure of the neurosurgeon to give the nurses sufficiently clear instructions and failure of the nurses to call the physician when the patient obviously was deteriorating. The jury returned a verdict of $700,000 against the hospital and the neurosurgeon.

Case 2

A 24-year-old woman had a therapeutic abortion. She was taken to the postoperative recovery room at 9:45 AM, where her blood pressure was noted to be 80/50. Her doctor checked her at that time and then left the hospital. A few minutes later, the patient's blood pressure was

70/40. At 10:10 AM, it was 64/60. The nurse telephoned the doctor, who said she told him the pulse was strong and that the patient seemed in good condition. Therefore, the doctor said he did not feel it was necessary to go to the hospital to evaluate the situation.

A few minutes later, the patient was taken to the intensive care unit, where her pressure was found to be 50/30. Her pulse was 88 and was characterized as "strong." The nurse's entries said the patient was "pale, alert, and responding."

The doctor was called again, but he later said that he was not given the sort of information that would have led him to conclude that there was an emergency. Therefore, instead of going to the hospital, which was only 5 minutes away, he told the nurse to call his associate, who was 30 minutes away. By the time the associate arrived, the patient was in shock. The defendant then came to the hospital and performed emergency surgery. The patient had experienced a massive hemorrhage into the broad ligament resulting from a perforated uterus with injury to the uterine artery. A cardiac arrest occurred midway through surgery. The patient's residual damage included hemiparesis with receptive and expressive aphasia. At trial, the physician testified that the nurse failed to characterize adequately the seriousness of the problem during each of her two calls. The result was a $1 million verdict against the hospital.

This case illustrates the importance of unambiguous communication. If the doctor does not respond appropriately, then the nurse must either persuade the doctor to act or obtain immediate assistance from another source. It is equally incumbent on physicians to ask the right questions to ensure that they have a full understanding of the situation.

THE TELEPHONE

Despite the sophisticated technology that is now integral to the practice of medicine, the humble telephone can be a dangerous instrument of professional liability. Telephone conversations are inherently deceptive because reliable communication requires facial expressions and body language to clarify what the voice is saying. Early morning phone conversations between weary attending physicians and hospital house officers are especially dangerous. Another hazardous situation arises in telephone communications with the ER. ER personnel usually have no prior knowledge of the patient and may have limited experience with the presenting condition. By offering medical advice on the phone, you can legally become the attending physician for a patient you have never seen. The following suggestions may help to protect you and your patients in this situation.

- Obtain as much information as possible about the patient.
- Prescribe or advise by phone only when you know the patient's medical history.
- Accept a third party's description of a medical condition only when you have confidence in that person's ability to accurately describe the situation and perform an appropriate evaluation.
- Do not hesitate to question the caller about his or her experience with a specific medical situation.
- Pursue any pertinent questions that are relevant to the medical problem.
- Insist on repetition of all vital instructions given to patients to ensure that they are clearly understood.
- Be especially wary of calls concerning abdominal or chest pain, fever, seizure, bleeding, head injury, dyspnea, a too-tight cast, neurologic alterations, or the onset of labor.
- Be certain that the pharmacist understands all dosages and instructions for drug prescriptions given by phone. Insist that the pharmacist recite the information back to you. Instruct your office personnel on the dangers of the automatic approval of prescription refills, even if they know a patient well. (The approval of certain prescriptions, such as analgesics, tranquilizers, antidepressants, or hormones, can prove hazardous without periodic examination.)
- If you take a call for another doctor, be especially on guard against telephone miscommunication. Do not make hasty decisions based solely on phone conversations. You may be held responsible for poor outcomes resulting from your telephone diagnosis.

The following cases are examples of serious consequences of poor telephone communication.

Case 1

Late one night, following a cervical laminectomy, a 52-year-old patient manifested bilateral grip weakness and tingling in his fingers. At 2 AM, the nurse telephoned an orthopedist who was on call for the patient's surgeon. The orthopedist had never seen the patient and later contended that he was not given a complete picture of the problem. Based on the assumption that the patient had ordinary complaints of pain, he gave the nurse routine analgesic orders. The patient's motor deficits continued and ultimately ended in quadraparesis. Although the orthopedist had never seen the patient, the court ruled that a doctor–patient relationship existed because the orthopedist had given orders. This case resulted in a $1.2 million verdict against the on-call doctor.

Faulty telephone communication between nurses and physicians is a vexing problem in malpractice suits because there is often disagreement about what was and was not said; sometimes there is poor documentation in the written medical record as well.

Case 2

A severely dehydrated 9-year-old girl suffering from viral gastroenteritis was admitted to a hospital pediatric ward at 5 AM. She was initially seen in the ER, but fluids had not been started. The ER physician admitted her and instructed the floor nurse to call the family physician. She did so, but there was a conflict in testimony concerning what was said.

The nurse contended that she had recounted the girl's vital signs and described her condition to the family doctor. However, the doctor testified that he was only told about the patient's complaint of abdominal pain and was not told of the severity of the dehydration. He ordered 50 mg of Demerol and a liter of 5% dextrose solution to be given intravenously.

Because of the hypovolemia, the nurse could not get an intravenous needle into the collapsed veins. However, she did not call the doctor again and the child's condition steadily worsened. At 9 AM, when the patient's doctor saw her, she was in profound shock. Despite appropriate treatment at that time, she died 3 hours later.

Case 3

A 38-year-old man had multiple leg fractures and a ruptured spleen as the result of an auto accident. Following stabilization of his leg fractures and a splenectomy, he developed shock lung syndrome. A nasotracheal tube was placed, and mechanical ventilation was initiated.

A few hours later, despite hand restraints, the patient pulled his tube out several inches, causing severe respiratory distress. The nurse came to the patient's bedside a few minutes after the incident and repositioned the tube. She then telephoned the general surgeon. The surgeon testified that the nurse failed to communicate the precise problem or its seriousness. The surgeon came to the hospital, but before doing so, he did not tell the nurse to remove the tube. He arrived just as the patient experienced a cardiac arrest, resulting in severe brain damage.

Case 4

An obstetrician called a colleague on a Friday afternoon to ask him if he would cover his patients for the weekend. He said he had only one patient who might deliver, but he failed to tell his colleague that a recent office examination indicated that there was a breech presentation. Early Sunday morning, the patient came to the hospital in labor, and the nurse failed to recognize the breech. At 5 AM, she telephoned the doctor, who gave routine orders and told her to call him back after labor progressed. The nurse was not especially attentive, until several hours later when she recognized a double footing breech presentation. The on-call doctor came to the hospital immediately, but there were serious problems with the birth and resuscitation. The result was a severely brain-damaged child. The doctor testified in deposition that had he known there was a breech presentation, he would have come to the hospital when he was first called. This was of little value after the fact.

CONCLUSION

Effective communication between physician and patient is probably the single most important element in the all-important equation we call doctor–patient rapport. Communication can be improved by following proven principles and techniques in both speaking and listening. Interactions among health care professionals can be equally problematic for different reasons but with devastating results. Much of the information transfer accepted as routine in medical practice is actually of potentially critical importance. It deserves the same focus and attention to process and outcome as other areas of medicine.

REFERENCES

1. Cassell EJ. Talking with Patients: Cambridge, MA: MIT Press, 1985.
2. Nichols RG. Are You Listening? New York, NY: McGraw Hill, 1957.
3. Morris D. Body Watching. New York, NY: Crown, 1985.
4. Morris D. Man Watching. New York, NY: Abrams, 1977.

7 E-Medicine in the Physician's Office

Edward Fotsch, MD

SUMMARY

E-medicine encompasses services including telephone, Internet, telemedicine, and electronic medical records. Each has unique potential to enhance the doctor–patient relationship and to increase physician liability. This chapter discusses each modality in detail. Detailed guidelines for online communication are presented.

Key Words: E-medicine; e-mail; risk reduction; telephone; online medical communication; Internet; guidelines for online communications; electronic medicine.

INTRODUCTION

E-medicine, or electronic medicine, refers to the use of electronic communication and information technology by physicians in the care of patients. Therefore, e-medicine encompasses various services including telephone, Internet, telemedicine, and electronic medical records. Each of these services has the unique potential to enhance the patient–physician relationship. As with all services that impact patient care, each also has the potential to increase physician liability.

From: *Medical Malpractice: A Physician's Sourcebook*
Edited by: R. E. Anderson © Humana Press Inc., Totowa, NJ

At the highest level, all forms of e-medicine share certain characteristics, as follow:

- Physicians are responsible for the services they provide for their patients.
- The appropriateness of the service and the potential value of the service will vary with specific patients.
- Appropriate patient expectations should be set.
- Standards of care or service, existing or evolving, should be followed to protect the interests of physicians and patients and to limit liability.
- Practical, financial, and technical considerations that impact the appropriate use of the service exist.
- Security and privacy considerations must be determined
- Record keeping should be an essential part of the service and an essential component of limiting physician liability.

The application of these principles varies with the specific service.

TELEPHONE-BASED CARE

The use of the telephone in the treatment of patients is neither new nor controversial. However, it does represent a legitimate form of patient care that has clear benefits as well as clear liabilities. When the telephone first emerged as a popular form of communication in the early 20th century, it was looked on with concern by many in the medical establishment. Warnings were given to doctors that the role of the telephone should not replace a face-to-face office visit and that telephone-based care could lead to suboptimal clinical outcomes and liability. Those concerns continue to be an issue.

Although the use of the telephone has become an essential component of medical care, particularly in the outpatient setting, it has largely been relegated to an administrative tool for setting appointments, refilling prescriptions, billing, and related administrative requests and questions. Physicians generally are not reimbursed for providing telephone-based care and, as the demands of physicians have increased with the advent of managed care, patient frustrations related to poor telephone access to their doctor has increased. Numerous national studies, including a national survey of patients done by Harris Polls, confirm growing patient frustration in their inability to communicate with their physicians via the telephone.

Telephone: Value and Appropriateness of the Service

It is hard to imagine running a physician's office without a telephone. Yet the use of the telephone varies widely among physicians, even within a single specialty. Some physicians are willing to spend large amounts of time on the phone with patients, whereas others rarely speak to patients outside of the exam room, opting instead to have most calls from patients returned by an office staff member. Whatever the protocol of the office, the physician is responsible for care delivered, regardless of whether it is delivered directly or through a member of the staff. In addition, the ability of a specific patient or caregiver to use telephone-based communication should be considered, as should the appropriateness of using the telephone to communicate sensitive clinical information.

Telephone: Patient Expectation

The growing frustration among patients regarding an inability to speak to their doctor on the phone only partially results from increased demands on the physician's time and a lack of reimbursement for telephone-based care. A substantial portion of this frustration stems from inadequate expectation management. It is guaranteed that patients or caregivers will want to telephone their doctor at some point, likely when a need arises and stress levels may be high. It is also guaranteed that doctors who spend entire days on the phone providing unreimbursed care to patients will quickly find their practices in financial trouble. The gap between patient expectation and practical limitations must be filled with disclosure and expectation management, preferably done ahead of the telephone ring, and in writing.

Physicians are well advised to develop written protocols associated with the appropriate use of the telephone in their practice. These protocols should be used to set patient expectations and to set office procedures that should be followed by all—physician and office staff alike. The procedures should be reviewed annually, and patients should be reminded of these protocols on a regular basis. The physician should consider posting protocols in areas where office staff has frequent access, as well as in employee handbooks. It is also advisable for the physician to be notified when and if a patient or caregiver has shown anger or frustration related to telephone-based communication. These concerns should be addressed by the physician and the practical and clinical issues associated with the office protocol should be reviewed directly with the patient.

Telephone: Standards of Care

The standards of care as they relate to telephone-based patient–physician communication do not vary significantly with specialty and practice setting. In all cases, the physician is held responsible for the adequacy and reasonableness of the communication. Most importantly, the physician must decide whether a face-to-face evaluation is necessary. The patient may be satisfied with a telephone consultation at the time, but if the outcome is adverse, the physician will need to be able to justify telephone-based care and not having insisted on a more direct intervention.

Telephone: Security and Privacy

Physicians are responsible for the appropriate security and privacy of their patients' records and information. Because the telephone has been in practical use by patients and physicians for decades, there are standard security and privacy technologies in place that provide safeguards. However, these safeguards are easily undermined by poor or unused protocols for the office. Physicians or staff can defeat standard safeguards, for example, by speaking on the phone with patients in a manner that allows unauthorized third parties to overhear the conversation. This potential for security breach, although rather obvious and theoretically simple to avoid, can become a practical challenge in the environment of a busy office setting. Well-defined procedures for telephone-based communication, including specific provisions to ensure patient privacy, will diminish potential risk.

The expansion of telephone-based communication to cell phones further expands the potential for security and privacy breach. The best approaches to diminishing these risks are to either avoid the use of cell phones for communication of patient information, or to consult the cell phone vendor about possible security breaches on the cell network. The potential risk from the use of cell phones can then be weighed against the practical need to use these networks. It is important to remember that the security concerns extend to the use of cell phones by patients as well as providers. The use of cell phones should be addressed in the office protocols. If appropriate, expectation setting should be done with patients relating to the use of cell phones, and appropriate disclaimers should be made.

Telephone: Practical/Technical/Financial Considerations

The practical and technical issues related to telephone-based care pale in comparison to the financial considerations. The plain facts are that the patient demand for telephone-based care, as experienced by most physicians, is very large, whereas the third-party payment for this care is nearly nonexistent. There is a Current Procedural Technology (CPT) code for telephone-based care, but few payors reimburse. Medicare, as a rule, does not reimburse for telephone-based care. Although some patients have expressed willingness to pay for the convenience of telephone-based care, most are not so willing. Physicians who have attempted to bill for telephone-based care have frequently been frustrated by the overhead associated with documenting the care and creating a patient invoice, and they are further frustrated by the poor collection rate and patient reaction to a fee-based telephone service. Because of this, many physicians have defaulted to a system of limited telephone-based care and look at the provision of this care as a cost-center for their practice. However, the financial realities of providing unreimbursed care must be weighed against the patient benefit of more convenient and more frequent access to their physician. Specifically, reimbursement policies cannot be allowed to limit necessary patient access. A phone call might be the first communication of an emergency or sentinel event signaling liability.

Telephone: Record Keeping

Clinically relevant care delivered via telephone should be documented in the patient's chart to fulfill state board, medical-legal, and standard-of-care requirements. This reality is made more challenging in that telephone-based care does not provide written documentation and physicians are not reimbursed for this documentation. Nonetheless, the documentation is required and poor documentation, as always, has the potential for profound liability ramifications. These protocols are especially important for "on-call" physicians or *locum tenens*.

INTERNET-BASED CARE

The growth of the Internet, websites, and e-mail has had a profound impact on health care and the practice of medicine, as it has on most other industries. However, health care has unique characteristics that strongly impact the manner in which the Internet is used. These include regulatory issues, such as the federal Health Insurance Portability and Accountability Act (HIPAA), liability issues, which will be discussed in more detail, and practical issues, such as the fact that most physicians are not employees and, therefore, decide with great independence whether they will use the Internet in the practice of medicine.

The Internet is rapidly working its way into the practice of medicine and will have profound impact on the patient–physician relationship.

Internet:
Physician Perspective

Many physicians now use e-mail regularly. An American Medical Association (AMA) survey in 2002 showed that nearly 90% of physicians are regular Internet users. The Internet has become an important means of both communication and professional education. In addition, nearly half of physicians have a website that is primarily used as a marketing vehicle to attract new patients to their practices. Although nearly 90% of physicians report regular e-mail use and nearly 50% report using e-mail to discuss patient care with other providers, only 25% report using e-mail with patients. A 2003 Harris Survey confirmed that physicians have three primary concerns regarding the use of e-mail with patients: payment, security, and liability. The survey also confirms continuing growth of e-mail in patient–physician communication, driven primarily by patient demand.

Professional associations, including the AMA and the American Academy of Physicians, have formally endorsed secure e-mail as an acceptable vehicle for ongoing patient care, albeit not for initiating a patient–physician relationship. Some health plans have started experimenting with payment for physician consultations provided online, further expanding the use of e-mail in the patient–physician relationship.

Internet:
Patient Expectation

According to the US Department of Commerce 2003 Survey, more than half of the US population now uses the Internet regularly, and households with a median income of $50,000 have a greater than 75% likelihood of being online. National surveys indicate that Internet use among those age 55 and older is one of the fastest growing age groups. Access to health care information and professional communication was noted by the federal government as a primary driver of Internet usage. Numerous national surveys, including the 2003 Harris survey of consumers, confirm that most patients want to be able to e-mail their doctors, and many are willing to change health plans or providers to gain e-mail access. In addition, nearly 40% of consumers who use the Internet regularly are willing to pay a fee to have e-mail access to their own doctor. Consumers point to the time and cost savings afforded by e-mail as the primary drivers of e-mail demand. With the growing shift of health care costs onto consumers, patient demand for e-mail access to their physicians is likely to grow.

Patient demand, or physician payment for online consultations, should not overshadow the need to use the Internet appropriately in patient–physician communication and to assess the individual patient's ability to use the service.

Internet:
Value and Appropriateness of the Service

The value of the Internet in the patient–physician relationship is only beginning to be quantified. However, it is clear that there are opportunities to enhance communication in a manner that promotes patient understanding as well as increasing communication efficiency. The "asynchronous" nature of e-mail and websites means that both the clinician and the patient can access and deliver information at a time and place that is convenient for him or her. This can be an important attribute to Internet-based communication, particularly when compared to the interruption and frustration that can be associated with ill-timed telephone calls or "telephone tag" between physicians and patients. It is also likely that providing patients with graphic instructions, available via websites, and a written record of physician instructions, via e-mail, can enhance the quality of patient understanding and provide an accurate document to which patients and care givers can refer repeatedly. E-mails can also be a vehicle to keep a dispersed group of family members and care givers "in sync" regarding a patient's care. The written record inherent in e-mail also can lead to enhanced physician record keeping and more thorough documentation, which is often critical in incidents of potential liability. Finally, Internet-based communication offers the ability to save and reuse quality clinical content through links to other websites or through the use of templates as the starting point for e-mail responses to frequently asked questions from patients.

However, patient–physician communication via the Internet is not a panacea and clearly has its limitations. The Internet is not an ideal communications vehicle to discuss highly sensitive or emergent matters. Complex matters such as a new diagnosis or a significant change in a patient's condition are not well-suited for e-mail. These limitations must be made clear to patients in a terms of service disclosure prior to initiating a substantive patient–physician relationship online.

An additional concern is the "digital divide," wherein many patients do not have access to or the ability to communicate via the Internet.

Although public libraries and other public venues may help, and more than half the US population now has Internet access in their homes, it does not necessarily follow that half of the patient population has ready Internet access or the ability to use the Internet.

Clinicians should carefully examine the benefits and limitations of Internet-based communication for themselves and for their patients, particularly in light of the increasing demand. A formal protocol should be established for the office and distributed to all staff and patients to set appropriate expectations. Whatever the protocol of the office, the physician is responsible for information and care delivered. Clinicians should also familiarize themselves with emerging state, federal, and industry regulations on the use of the Internet in patient–physician communication.

Internet:
Standards of Care, Security, and Privacy

As use of the Internet becomes more common in the delivery of health care, standards of online care and service arise. Some are dictated through legislation, such as the HIPAA statute enacted by the federal government. State medical boards also will play a role in setting and enforcing regulations. Indeed, several state boards have already taken disciplinary action against practioners who have violated state board regulations related to online patient–physician interaction. These punitive actions have focused on the provision of care and the delivery of prescriptions when there is no pre-existing relationship between the physician and the patient. The need for a previously established patient–physician relationship is commonly recognized as a requirement in care delivered online.

However, there are other generally accepted standards that go beyond government legislation and extend to generally accepted standards of care. As is the case in most of medical practice, norms and guidelines for standard of care evolve from medical organizations, liability carriers, medical societies, and state medical boards. Fortunately for practicing physicians, these four entities have found a forum, the "eRisk Working Group," to work together to create a single set of guidelines for clinicians as they communicate with patients in an online environment.

The eRisk Guidelines have been developed by the eRisk Working Group for Health Care, a consortium of professional liability carriers, medical societies, and state board representatives. These guidelines are meant to provide information to health care providers related to online communication. They are reviewed and updated regularly. These guidelines are not meant as legal advice, and providers are encouraged to bring any specific questions or issues related to online communication to their legal counsel.

ONLINE COMMUNICATIONS ERISK GUIDELINES

The legal rules, ethical guidelines, and professional etiquette that govern and guide traditional communications between the health care provider and patient are equally applicable to e-mail, websites, listservs, and other electronic communications.

However, the technology of online communications introduces special concerns and risks. The following lists some of the concerns involved in online communication:

1. Security

    Online communications between health care provider and patient should be conducted over a secure network, with provisions for authentication and encryption in accordance with eRisk, HIPAA, and other appropriate guidelines. Standard e-mail services do not meet these guidelines. Health care providers need to be aware of potential security risks, including unauthorized physical access and security of computer hardware, and guard against them with technologies such as automatic logout and password protection.

2. Authentication

    The health care provider has a responsibility to take reasonable steps to authenticate the identity of correspondent(s) in an electronic communication and to ensure that recipients of information are authorized to receive it.

3. Confidentiality

    The health care provider is responsible for taking reasonable steps to protect patient privacy and to guard against unauthorized use of patient information.

4. Unauthorized Access

    The use of online communications may increase the risk of unauthorized distribution of patient information and create a clear record of this distribution. Health care providers should establish and follow procedures that help to mitigate this risk.

5. Informed Consent

    Prior to the initiation of online communication between health care provider and patient, informed consent should be obtained from the patient regarding the appropriate use and limitations of this form of communication. Providers should consider developing and publishing specific guidelines for online communications with patients, such as avoiding emergency use, heightened consideration of use for highly sensitive medical topics, appropriate expectations for response times, and so forth. These guidelines should become part of the legal documentation and medical record when appropriate. Providers should consider developing patient selection criteria to identify those patients suitable for e-mail correspondence, thus eliminating persons who would not be compliant.

6. Highly Sensitive Subject Matter

The health care provider should advise patients of potential privacy risks associated with online communication related to highly sensitive medical subjects. This warning should be repeated if a provider solicits information of a highly sensitive nature, such as issues of mental health, substance abuse, and so forth. Providers should avoid active initial solicitation of highly sensitive topic matters.

7. Emergency Subject Matter

The health care provider should advise patients of the risks associated with online communication related to emergency medical subjects such as chest pain, shortness of breath, bleeding during pregnancy, and so forth. Providers should avoid active promotion of the use of online communication to address topics of medical emergencies.

8. Doctor–Patient Relationship

The health care provider may increase liability exposure by initiating a doctor–patient relationship solely through online interaction. Payment for online services may further increase that exposure.

9. Medical Records

Whenever possible and appropriate, a record of online communications pertinent to the ongoing medical care of the patient must be maintained as part of, and integrated into, the patient's medical record, whether that record is paper or electronic.

10. Licensing Jurisdiction

Online interactions between a health care provider and a patient are subject to requirements of state licensure. Communications online with a patient outside of the state in which the provider holds a license may subject the provider to increased risk.

11. Authoritative Information

Health care providers are responsible for the information that they provide or make available to their patients online. Information that is provided on a medical practice website should come either directly from the health care provider or from a recognized and credible source. Information provided to specific patients via secure e-mail from a health care provider should come either directly from the health care provider or from a recognized and credible source after review by the provider.

12. **Commercial Information**
Websites and online communications of an advertising, promotional, or marketing nature may subject providers to increased liability, including implicit guarantees or implied warranty. Misleading or deceptive claims increase this liability.

FEE-BASED ONLINE CONSULTATIONS eRISK GUIDELINES

A fee-based online consultation is a clinical consultation provided by a medical provider to a patient using the Internet or other similar electronic communications network in which the provider expects payment for the service.

An online consultation that is given in exchange for payment introduces additional risks. In a fee-based online consultation, the healthcare provider has the same obligations for patient care and follow-up as in face-to-face, written, and telephone consultations. For example, an online consultation should include an explicit follow-up plan that is clearly communicated to the patient.

In addition to the 12 guidelines stated earlier, the following are additional considerations for fee-based online consultations:

1. **Pre-Existing Relationship**
Online consultations should occur only within the context of a previously established doctor–patient relationship that includes a face-to-face encounter when clinically appropriate. State medical boards have begun enforcement actions.

2. **Informed Consent**
Prior to the online consultation, the health care provider must obtain the patient's informed consent to participate in the consultation for a fee. The consent should include explicitly stated disclaimers and service terms pertaining to online consultations. The consent should establish appropriate expectations between provider and patient.

3. **Medical Records**
Records pertinent to the online consultation must be maintained as part of, and integrated into, the patient's medical record.

4. **Fee Disclosure**
From the outset of the online consultation, the patient must be clearly informed about charges that will be incurred and that the charges may not be reimbursed by the patient's health insurance. If the patient chooses not to participate in the fee-based consultation, the patient should be encouraged to contact the provider's office by phone or other means.

5. Appropriate Charges

An online consultation should be substantive and clinical in nature and be specific to the patient's personal health status. There should be no charge for online administrative or routine communications such as appointment scheduling and prescription refill requests. Health care providers should consider not charging for follow-up questions on the same subject as the original online consultation.

6. Identity Disclosure

Clinical information that is provided to the patient during the course of an online consultation should come from, or be reviewed in detail by, the consulting provider, whose identity should be made clear to the patient.

7. Available Information

Health care providers should state, within the context of the consultation, that it is based only on information made available by the patient to the provider during or prior to the online consultation, including referral to the patient's chart when appropriate and, therefore, may not be an adequate substitute for an office visit.

8. Online Consultation vs Online Diagnosis and Treatment

Health care providers should attempt to distinguish between online consultation related to pre-existing conditions, ongoing treatment, follow-up question related to previously discussed conditions, and so forth, and new diagnosis and treatment addressed solely online. New diagnosis and treatment of conditions, solely online, may increase liability exposure.

The following copyright information is provided to users of the guidelines:

Copyright © 2002 Medem, Inc. Used with the permission of Medem, Inc. and the eRisk Working Group for Health care.

As patient–physician communication online expands, the standards of care and service will evolve. It is conceivable that, in the not-too-distant future, the use of online communication will become as commonplace as the use of the telephone and there will be generally accepted norms for availability of clinicians to patients. For the time being, clinicians are encouraged to err on the side of discretion, disclosure, and prudence in delivering care online to their patients. Clinicians are also warned to keep accurate records of online communication with and about patients, because these records are now routinely subpoenaed in liability litigation. Clinicians must show the same accuracy and discretion in online patient communication, as they would in any written clinical document.

Internet:
Practical/Technical/Financial Considerations

The practical and technical issues related to Internet-based care are now being resolved. Internet access is nearly ubiquitous in the United States, even in physician's offices, and nearly all educated Americans are able to efficiently use e-mail and the Web. Inexpensive high-speed Internet connections are becoming the norm and the cost of access is decreasing. Wireless Internet communication is rapidly expanding, further lowering costs and barriers to instantaneous and ubiquitous online access. The greatest practical concerns among clinicians related to online patient–physician communication are security/liability issues and the fear of additional hours spent in unreimbursed patient care. The former issues have been largely addressed through legislation and industry adoption of guidelines and standards of care. The financial concerns can be addressed as well through the delivery of fee-based online consultations, wherein the patient pays a nominal fee, typically commensurate with a health plan copayment, to access his or her physician through the convenience of an online interactive session. There is a CPT code for online consultations, but few payors are presently reimbursing for this service.

Clinicians can make online interactions with patients even more efficient by using templates as a starting point for frequently asked questions. Online communication creates an automatic record of the patient–clinician communication that can be saved electronically or in print. However, physicians are cautioned to write, review, and/or edit all information that goes to a patient in an online communication under the physician's name and to save all communication, particularly in the case of fee-based online consultations. Again, disclosure and transparency for the patient, and careful record keeping is essential.

8 Risk Management for the Family Physician

Malcolm H. Weiss, MD

SUMMARY

This chapter focuses on legal, clinical, and risk-management issues that create pitfalls for the family physician. Examples of legal issues are vicarious liability and ostensible agency. Clinical issues include the timely diagnosis and treatment of conditions such as cancer and heart disease. Difficult-to-diagnose conditions such as pulmonary emboli and dissecting aortic aneurysms are also discussed. Risk-management issues that can destroy an otherwise viable defense are also noted. These include record tampering, failure to obtain informed consent or informed refusal, and the practice of treating patients over the telephone. The importance of the contemporaneous medical record is stressed.

Key Words: Risk management; informed consent; record tampering; standard of care; prescription errors.

INTRODUCTION

Failure to consider the medical-legal context in which medicine is practiced can undermine the defensibility of good medicine. Consider the case of a middle-aged man who was diagnosed by his family physician with chest wall pain and was treated conservatively. He died a

From: *Medical Malpractice: A Physician's Sourcebook*
Edited by: R. E. Anderson © Humana Press Inc., Totowa, NJ

few days later with an autopsy-confirmed massive myocardial infarction. A lawsuit was filed. Failure to diagnose coronary artery disease was alleged. The family physician reviewed his office record and panicked. There were hints in the chief complaint and history of present illness that suggested heart disease. The family physician altered the original chart entry. A suspicious plaintiff's attorney sent the chart to a laboratory that specialized in detecting record tampering. The lab was able to prove that the record had been altered. Medical care that might have been considered appropriate by a reasonable jury was now clouded by a physician who had lost all credibility. The case was settled for an amount in excess of the policy limit.

Generally speaking, medical malpractice lawsuits are based on allegations of clinical error, medical-legal error, or combinations of the two. This chapter addresses both.

The case just presented is a clear example of a medical-legal error. Had the defendant physician paid heed to the warnings that all physicians receive regarding the alteration of records, he would have avoided an emotionally draining and costly experience.

GENERAL ISSUES AND CONSIDERATIONS

The malpractice crisis is forever upon us. Family physicians continually work under the threat of litigation. In addition, there is the threat of regulatory sanction for Occupational Safety and Health Administration, Clinical Laboratory Improvement Act, and Health Insurance Portability and Accountability Act violations. There are also penalties for Medicare and Medicaid violations. Private insurers and managed care organizations put additional pressure on physicians. It seems as though family physicians live their entire professional lives under a microscope. The stresses under which they live and work direct their attention away from clinical medicine and increase the chance for error.

Family practice is a specialty in breadth rather than depth. Its responsibilities cross almost all other specialty lines. As gatekeepers, family physicians are expected to make the correct diagnosis in a cost-effective manner. As referring physicians, they are expected to make timely referrals to appropriate specialists. As treating physicians, they are held to the standards of each relevant specialty.

UNFORESEEN LEGAL PITFALLS

Under the doctrine of vicarious liability, a family physician can be held liable for the actions of another physician when a patient reasonably believes that there is a financial or professional relationship between them. Independent physicians who share waiting rooms or office space are at risk. To avoid misunderstandings, physicians in these situations should make their independence clear to patients. A clearly written statement signed by the patient may prevent future litigation.

California law (Civil Code Section 2300) states that ostensible agency occurs "when the principal intentionally, or by want of ordinary care, causes a third party to believe another to be his agent who is not really employed by him." Other states have similar provisions. It is important for family physicians to seek the advice of their attorneys to avoid the trap of ostensible agency.

STANDARD-OF-CARE CONCERNS

The challenge created by the accelerating rate of medical advance is especially relevant to primary care physicians. Patients expect them to be aware of new diagnostic and treatment modalities. The family physician is required to meet the standard of care regarding each patient. However, the standard of care is not formally recorded anywhere. It is usually defined as that which a competent physician would do under the same circumstances. It is significant that the competent physician need not be in the same specialty or in the same community as the family physician in question. Therefore, it is incumbent on the family physician to be both up to date and to know his or her limitations. Family physicians must take continuing medical education seriously. They must read respected medical journals. Three that are frequently cited in litigation are *American Family Physician*, *The Journal of the American Medical Association*, and *The New England Journal of Medicine*.

ALLEGATION CONCERNS

Many physicians are intimidated by the increasing number of rules, regulations, and potential penalties thrust on them. Plaintiff attorneys are very innovative. There is no end to the number of new physician responsibilities they devise. To make matters worse, "hired guns," physicians who will testify to anything for a price, are always a threat. It is important for the physician to be an active member of the medical community by taking advantage of the expertise offered by county, state, and national medical societies; and by participating in hospital staff proceedings. As a defendant in a medical malpractice suit, the physician must work very closely with his or her insurer and defense attorney.

All materials in the claim file should be read carefully. "Hired guns" may not only fabricate and misquote but also may sign affidavits or reports written by the plaintiff attorney without reading them. Helping one's defense attorney discredit a hired gun can lead to a verdict for the defense.

RULES TO BE OBEYED

"First do no harm" is a rule as old as the practice of medicine itself. Equally important is the rule that the dignity of the patient must be preserved. Physicians who fail to abide by these rules may find themselves defendants in indefensible lawsuits. For example, there is the case of an educated woman who presented to her physician with a chief complaint of rectal bleeding. A nurse practitioner diagnosed a resolving external hemorrhoid without performing a rectal examination or any other diagnostic procedure. The patient returned 1 year later with the same complaint. The physician saw her. The same diagnosis was made. It is documented in the record that the patient requested sigmoidoscopy. Her request was denied. Several months later, a gastroenterologist diagnosed rectal carcinoma. The case was settled in favor of the plaintiff.

In another case, a primary care physician performed a carpal tunnel release in his office without prior training. The median nerve was severed. The patient suffered permanent disability. This case was also settled in favor of the plaintiff.

In the rectal carcinoma case, the patient was harmed by the physician's failure to supervise the nurse practitioner and to appropriately evaluate the patient's complaint. Her dignity was not preserved. She was treated with disrespect when her reasonable request for an indicated procedure was denied.

In the second case, an untrained physician harmed the patient. The patient was disrespected when his right to skilled care was disregarded.

The increasing incidence of plaintiff demands for punitive damages should be taken seriously. Physicians who permit themselves or members of their staff to act in an unprofessional manner or who fail to insist on the professional appearance of their office or clinic show disrespect for the dignity of the patient. Physicians who perform procedures for which they are not appropriately trained not only show disrespect but also risk doing harm. Physicians who bill insurers for visits never made or bill for more intense levels of service than the severity of the illness calls for devalue their patients. Patients treated in such an underhanded manner will sue at the slightest provocation.

PHYSICIAN EXTENDERS

Rules regarding physician extenders need to be understood. Individual state laws must be obeyed. Patient safety is a paramount consideration. Physician extenders must be clearly identified. Their training, skills, and responsibilities must be disclosed. The responsibilities of the supervising physician must be understood. Patient preferences must be respected.

There is a case involving a mother who brought a sick infant to a clinic. A professional appearing gentleman wearing a white lab coat saw the patient. His nameplate had the initials "PA" (physician's assistant) after his name. The mother was not told that he was not a physician or that a physician would not see her baby. The diagnosis of meningitis was missed. The infant died and litigation followed.

DIFFERENTIAL DIAGNOSIS

Rules regarding differential diagnosis need to be defined. Differential diagnosis is not an academic exercise. It is a clinically significant documentation of the physician's thinking. When a physician writes "chest wall pain, rule out myocardial ischemia" or "gastroenteritis, rule out appendicitis," potentially life-threatening entities must be ruled out before the patient is permitted to leave the site. Failure to do so may lead to the patient's death.

The more common of the life-threatening entities should be recorded. The esoteric diagnosis need not be recorded initially. A carefully thought out history and physical will guide the physician. If the more common entities are ruled out, then additional diagnostic possibilities should be considered. In the case of chest wall pain, historical facts may make it necessary to first rule out myocardial ischemia, pleurisy, and pulmonary emboli. As new information is gathered, it may become necessary to rule out dissecting thoracic aortic aneurysm, metastatic cancer, herpes zoster, and so on. In today's world of cost containment and cost-effective medicine, a logical sequential approach to differential diagnosis should be employed and documented. However, time is of the essence.

CLINICAL ISSUES

The following is a list of clinical issues that are the most common causes of claims against family physicians:

1. Cancer: diagnosis and treatment.
2. Heart disease: prevention, diagnosis, and treatment.

3. Acute surgical abdomen: timely diagnosis and timely referral to a surgical specialist.
4. Diabetes: early diagnosis, treatment, and prevention of complications.
5. Pneumonia: early diagnosis, treatment, and timely referral when appropriate.

In addition to these, the following are the most common specific entities that create major diagnostic and treatment pitfalls for primary care physicians:

1. Pulmonary emboli.
2. Atypical angina pectoris.
3. Dissecting aortic aneurysm: those involving the thoracic aorta are often misdiagnosed.
4. Meningitis: patients of all ages are involved. Failure to diagnose in small children has led to tragedy and many lawsuits.
5. Antibiotic-resistant infections: these are a major concern for hospitalized and nursing home patients.
6. Pain: failure to recognize and appropriately manage pain is not only a breach of the standard of care but is also grounds for allegations of abuse and requests for punitive damages. Allegations of elder abuse are very common when caregivers believe that pain is not being responsibly treated.

In the case of these six entities, a high index of suspicion is necessary to make the proper diagnosis in a timely manner. Death from a pulmonary embolus usually results from failure to diagnose rather than failure to treat. There are no specific symptoms, but there are risk factors. There are also new diagnostic tools. Once pulmonary embolus is suspected, timely intervention and consultation with appropriate specialists can be life-saving.

By definition, atypical angina pectoris needs to be suspected before it can be diagnosed. It is also important to consider recent studies that conclude that many women with coronary artery disease do not present with chest pain. Their presenting complaints often are fatigue and insomnia.

The most common location for the pain of a dissecting aortic aneurysm is the precordium. The sudden onset of a tearing pain between the shoulder blades need not be present. The possibility of this diagnosis should be kept in mind when an acute myocardial infarction is suspected. A normal electrocardiogram and normal enzymes can help differentiate the two. Bear in mind that the two entities can coexist. A timely consultation will benefit both the patient and the family physician.

Meningitis, especially in small children, is a diagnostic challenge. Pediatric textbooks describe the usual and the atypical presentations. It is advisable to consider meningitis in an infant that is febrile, lethargic, and anorexic. When it is reasonable to suspect meningitis, a lumbar puncture is mandatory.

Antibiotic-resistant infections, such as those caused by methicillin-resistant staph aureus, plague patients in hospitals and nursing homes. The effects can be devastating. They often lead to sepsis, septic shock, organ failure, and death. When the elderly are involved, there are not only allegations of malpractice but also of elder abuse. In this case, punitive damages, which are not covered by insurance, may be awarded. It is necessary for family physicians to be informed of hospital and skilled nursing facility nosocomial infection experience and to demand that all appropriate preventative measures are taken. Principles regarding culture and sensitivity studies and consultation with infectious disease and surgical specialists should be followed.

Pain management presents many pitfalls for primary care physicians. Physicians walk a fine line between prescribing too much and too little. Often, allegations of negligence and abuse are made after the patient is deceased. Some patients prefer to tolerate pain to remain alert. Their wishes must be documented and witnessed by a family member or a caregiver, such as a nurse. In problem situations, consultation with a pain management specialist may be necessary.

There is no way to completely avoid allegations of failure to meet the standard of care in each of the aforementioned clinical matters. However, family physicians can create defensive postures that will make them difficult targets. First, continuing medical education in relevant areas should be documented. For example, proof that a physician has successfully completed a recent American Medical Association- or American Academy of Family Physicians-accredited course in pain management can be very helpful to the defense when the allegation is failure to manage pain appropriately. Second, it should be documented that accepted diagnostic and treatment protocols have been followed. Third, physicians should avoid the appearance of getting in over their heads by referring in a timely manner. Fourth, one should pay attention to concerns of nurses, technicians, physician extenders, and family members. Physicians should show that they care. Finally, it must be remembered that physicians are patient advocates. Third-party delays or failure to approve are not excuses for denying patients needed care in a timely manner. Aggressive advocacy should be taken for all patients.

RISK-MANAGEMENT ISSUES

One of the most serious risk-management allegations made against family physicians is failure to obtain informed consent. The patient or the patient's guardian has the right to know all of the information that a reasonable person would need to make an intelligent decision. It is the physician's duty to provide the information in a manner that is understandable to the recipient. This is best documented by a signed and witnessed informed consent form. The exact nature of the form depends on individual state law. It is best for physicians to use forms that have passed legal scrutiny by their state.

Informed consent is not only necessary for invasive procedures but also for examination, diagnostic tests, treatment modalities, and prescribed medication. The following list contains information that should appear in all informed consent forms.

1. The diagnosis.
2. The nature and purpose of the proposed test, examination, or treatment.
3. Risks, including possible side effects or complications, as well as benefits.
4. The probability of success as well as failure.
5. Alternatives.
6. The consequences of doing nothing or of seeking alternatives that are not advised.
7. The consequences of delay.

Although informed consent will not protect a physician from all charges of professional negligence, it is important to address the most common and most serious risks of a procedure. Colonoscopy presents a good example. Risks to be noted are infection, bleeding, colon perforation, peritonitis, and sepsis. Also to be noted is the risk of missing a small but significant lesion. What will a family physician do if spasm or obstruction prevents a complete examination? Patients have the right to know.

There is also the duty to obtain informed refusal. In 1980, the California Supreme Court (27 CAL. 3d 285) established this doctrine when it ruled for the plaintiff in the case of a woman who died of advanced cervical cancer. Her family physician's record documented that over a period of years he had repeatedly advised a routine Pap smear. However, the record did not establish that he had ever explained the reason for a Pap smear or the potential risks of not having one. The patient's family was able to successfully argue that if she had known that the purpose of a Pap smear was to detect cervical cancer, then she might have given consent.

A surgeon severed a major nerve while performing surgery for squamous cell carcinoma. The patient suffered postoperative disability. A lawsuit followed. In his defense, the surgeon claimed that the nerve was so matted down in the tumor that it had to be sacrificed for a complete excision. Unfortunately, the surgeon dictated a generic operative note that made no mention of a difficult dissection. There is a rule in risk management that if it is not documented, then it did not happen. The jury awarded a large sum to the plaintiff.

There is an interesting side issue in this case. The possibility of severing the nerve was not mentioned in the informed consent document. However, failure to obtain informed consent was not an issue. The incident occurred in a state that requires an objective standard for informed consent. The plaintiff would have had to show that with full disclosure, a reasonable patient would have rejected the procedure. The consequences of rejecting this surgery would have been devastating, far outweighing the consequences of a severed nerve. A reasonable patient would opt for the surgery. Many states adhere to this objective standard. Other states adhere to a subjective standard meaning that only the decision of the patient in question is considered. It is advisable for physicians to seek the opinion of an attorney in their own state regarding objective and subjective standards for informed consent.

Altering medical records can destroy an otherwise viable defense. Jurors rely heavily on the reliability of contemporaneous medical records. Altered records destroy a physician's credibility. Any change, even when initialed and dated, can be made to appear self-serving. Concerns should be discussed with the defense attorney. Records should always be left alone.

Almost as damaging as an altered record is an ambiguous one. For example, a young woman suffered from metastatic breast cancer. After surgery, but prior to the discovery of metastases, a panel of experts recommended a course of chemotherapy. The patient's physician was aware of the experts' advice. However, the patient never received chemotherapy. She sued after being diagnosed with widespread metastases. The office record was not clear that the patient had been informed about the recommendation for chemotherapy. The patient stated that she would have accepted the risks to have more time to spend with her family if she had been given the choice. The case was settled for a large sum.

We advise the use of the SOAP format for documentation of physician–patient encounters. SOAP is an acronym for subjective, objective, assessment, and plan—the patient's *subjective* complaints, the physician's *objective* findings, the physician's *assessment*, and his or her *plan* for evaluation and management. This format has been taught in medical schools for more than 20 years. It allows the physician to organize his or her thoughts and document an approach that is best suited for the care of the patient. Had the physician in the case just described documented his assessment and plan, he would have avoided a costly malpractice suit.

Every physician's office or clinic should have a fail-safe system in place to ensure that every report, indeed every patient-related scrap of paper, must be read and initialed by a physician before being added to a patient's chart. Recommendations by other health care providers must be acted on. The decision to wait, to observe, or to repeat an evaluation is acceptable as long as it is documented and explained. Members of large groups who rotate through satellite offices have an extra burden in this regard. Court documents describe many cases where elevated prostate-specific antigens and other lab tests, abnormal pathology reports, mammograms, X-rays, and so on are filed without being reviewed by a physician. Months to years later, metastatic cancer is diagnosed. It is alleged that had the original report been acted on, the cancer would have been diagnosed at a time when a cure was possible. This is a difficult argument to refute, especially to a public trained in the value of early detection and in the face of a clear breach in the standard of care.

The Telephone

A major pitfall for physicians is treating patients over the telephone. This is often necessary and appropriate. However, the doctor must be satisfied that he or she has gathered all the necessary information and the patient understands the recommendation and the need for follow-up. In addition, it is critical that telephone conversations be documented and entered into the medical record. This is especially important when medication is prescribed. It is also necessary to inform the attending physician of any actions or encounters that occur in the on-call setting. Too often, malpractice suits hinge on a credibility test between the memory of the physician and the testimony of the patient. When there is any doubt, the doctor should meet the patient in the emergency room for a formal evaluation. A famous plaintiff attorney once stated that he would never have a problem earning a good living by suing doctors as long as they persisted in the "stupidity" of treating patients over the telephone.

Prescription Errors

These are a common source of litigation for family physicians. Prescriptions must be clearly written. There are so many instances of patients receiving Purinethol when propylthiouracil was prescribed that in June 2003, GlaxoSmithKline sent health care professionals a "Medication Errors Alert," warning of the consequences of this error. Patients must be well-informed regarding the drugs they are prescribed. It is a good idea to include the indication on the prescription so that a patient does not inadvertently take an antibiotic in place of an antihypertensive, for example. Because Purinethol has its name imprinted on every tablet, an informed patient would not take the wrong drug.

Patients need to be alerted about other look-alike and sound-alike medications. They should also be alerted regarding correct dosages, allergies, side effects, and the appropriate use of controlled substances. Informed consent is required and should be documented, especially for drugs that may have serious side effects. Excessive prescribing and inappropriate use of prescription drugs are grounds for malpractice suits as well as loss of prescribing privileges and suspension or loss of a medical license.

Refill practices must be clearly defined for the benefit of patients and pharmacists. Prescriptions must be legible. The patient must understand the physician's refill instructions. The pharmacist must understand the physician's policy concerning controlled substances. Steps must be taken to prevent hoarding and then overdosing at a later date. The patient must understand in advance the physician's policy regarding lost prescriptions and drugs destroyed by the dog or flushed down the toilet or stolen from a woman's purse. Some drugs that patients are permitted to refill require close monitoring. Examples are Coumadin and drugs that treat diabetes. If a patient fails to comply with monitoring instructions, the privilege to refill may have to be withdrawn. Finally, there must be systems in place to warn patients of drug recalls. Rezulin, Seldane, and Baycol are good examples.

Procedures

It is clearly a breach of the standard of care for physicians or their assistants to perform procedures for which they are not adequately trained. Melanomas have been incompletely excised by unskilled physicians. In one case, a woman's face was badly scarred by a physician who was trained in the use of a laser by a salesperson. The physician's prior experience involved an orange. Botox injections have caused nerve damage. Unskilled endoscopists have perforated organs. Soft tissue injections around the scapula or into an intercostal muscle have perforated lungs. Joint injections by those not properly trained have caused destructive septic arthritis. These and similar misadventures have led to lawsuits that are very difficult to defend.

The Language Barrier

The problems related to language barriers are well known to physicians. Patients with limited English skills cannot be denied health care or in any way be discriminated against by health care providers. In 2000, President Clinton issued Executive Order 13166, requiring equal access to federally funded health care services for patients with limited English proficiency. A language barrier will probably not shield a physician from allegations of negligence. In one recent case, a physician failed to diagnose a subarachnoid hemorrhage because he could not understand the history of onset or severity of a headache. A patient who is not proficient in English cannot be ignored. There are different types of aids available. Interpreters on the telephone or, better still, in the office are invaluable. Before discharging a patient, a physician should be certain that he or she understands the medical problems and that the patient understands the necessary advice and follow-up.

SUMMATION

At any given time, 15–20% of physicians are defendants in malpractice lawsuits. The average lawsuit takes more than 3 years from inception to resolution. The experience can destroy a physician's health, family relationships, standing in the community, self-confidence, and financial security. There have even been suicides where objective evaluation indicated that the physician was not guilty of wrongdoing. Risk managers have been criticized for advising strategies that are too time-consuming. Yet, when considering the alternatives, they may be time well spent. The future is uncertain. New laws, rules, and court decisions continue to create additional responsibilities and risks for physicians. Physicians are best advised to anticipate and prepare for change.

Finally, it should be kept in mind that a family physician's best friends in a malpractice lawsuit are the contemporaneous, thoughtful, clearly written medical record and a supportive, competent, caring nurse. Neither should be tampered with.

9 Emergency Medicine

Michael Jay Bresler, MD, FACEP

SUMMARY

This chapter reviews some general medical and legal principles, most of which are important regardless of medical specialty. They are particularly relevant to emergency physicians but are also important to physicians from other specialties who treat patients in the emergency department (ED). I then discuss some specific emergency medical conditions that often result in litigation. The topics presented are not meant to be an exhaustive list of potential liability problems, but rather a sample of some of the more common issues that confront physicians and their patients.

Key Words: Emergency; emergency medicine; emergency department; medical-legal; risk management.

INTRODUCTION

Emergency medicine is a very enjoyable specialty. Emergency physicians revel in the excitement, chaos, and challenge presented by emergency patients. Basically, we are action junkies. And we like the unknown.

Most of the time, our patients appreciate our efforts. Unfortunately, we are also appreciated by another class of people—plaintiff attorneys. They like us precisely because we practice in a hectic, somewhat

From: *Medical Malpractice: A Physician's Sourcebook*
Edited by: R. E. Anderson © Humana Press Inc., Totowa, NJ

uncontrolled environment in which we confront complex problems in a limited, and usually rushed, time frame. They like us because our patients often are either very ill or will become very ill. And they like us because they know that we cannot always predict which of our patients will become very ill or die in the near future. In short, we are often cannon fodder for our legal brethren.

Although we will be emphasizing the avoidance of liability, remember that the best defense, as is often said, is to do the right thing. Our goal is not just to avoid being sued, it is to practice the best quality medicine of which we are capable for our own sake and, most importantly, for the sake of our patients.

GENERAL PRINCIPLES: WE (SHOULD) HOLD THESE TRUTHS TO BE SELF-EVIDENT

Communication Is Crucial

Let the patient speak. Let the family speak. One of the most common complaints of patients filing lawsuits is that they felt the doctor was not really interested in them. The doctor would not let them fully present their problem, and quickly cut them off. This is a real possibility, particularly in the emergency department (ED). We are usually quite pressed for time and, as we all know, patients can be rather verbose. Many give the impression that they rather enjoy regaling doctors with their tales of woe. And patients often do not understand what is relevant to us and to their acute problems vs what is more related to their chronic conditions.

Sometimes, we have to limit the patient's free speech. However, I would suggest first giving patients 1 or 2 minutes to expound before zeroing in on the problem. Try not to interrupt too soon. Allow patients to ventilate. Usually, they are truly worried about their health, and merely discussing the problem with a caring physician is somewhat therapeutic. Besides, you never know what you'll learn! You may know more about the medical problem than they do, but they know more about their own symptoms.

Families are also important. Obviously, there are some social and/ or medical conditions that demand privacy. At times, it is appropriate to ask a family member or friend to leave the room. Potential Ob/Gyn problems are typical of this situation. However, I would suggest having the family in the room when appropriate. It usually increases the patient's comfort level, especially during long waits in the sterile and somewhat intimidating environment of the examining room.

More importantly, family members often provide crucial information. We've all heard the wife tell us that her husband is downplaying his symptoms. He's actually had chest pain off and on for 3 days, not just for 2 minutes. If there is any question of altered level of consciousness or abnormal behavior, then the observations of the family or friends may be absolutely crucial.

Lack of English Is No Excuse—for You

The law says it is our fault if a language barrier interferes with communication. We are a nation of immigrants. All of us, or our ancestors, came from somewhere else, even Native Americans. Immigrants often do not have insurance and they are disproportionately represented among our patients in the ED.

There is not only a language variation but a cultural variation as well. Different cultures allow people to express pain differently. Some cultures seem to encourage demonstrative behavior with illness. Others encourage stoicism. Depending on the background of the physician, we may be misled by these cultural differences.

In some cultures, it is deemed disrespectful to let the doctor think you do not understand him or her. The patient may be embarrassed by lack of English facility. Perhaps you have had the experience of asking the patient if he or she understands what you're saying, and he or she nods yes. You then ask if he or she is totally confused, and he or she nods yes again. Were you to ask if the patient was eaten by a horse, you may receive another nod yes. By this time, it may occur to you that you have a language as well as a cultural problem.

Ideally, use of an interpreter is best. However, AT&T provides a 24-hour foreign-language hotline that can be extremely helpful if you do not have an interpreter available. This service is available for a multitude of foreign languages. Trained volunteers speak by phone with both the physician and the patient, and I have found this service to be excellent. You might consider installing a phone with two handsets so that you can both speak with the interpreter simultaneously.

A family member may be used to interpret when appropriate. However, be aware of socially sensitive situations, particularly regarding Ob/Gyn issues.

Document

Document. Document. Document. And one more thing: Document! In legal proceedings such as depositions and in court, a stenographer records every single word spoken; nowadays, stenographers use tape recorders and computerized stenographs. Obviously, we do not have such luxuries in the ED.

Nevertheless, the eternal truth according to plaintiff attorneys is as follows: "If it wasn't documented, it wasn't done." Physicians know this is nonsense, but do not give them the opportunity to argue it. Document pertinent positives and pertinent negatives. It will not be sufficient in front of a jury to say that you did not document pertinent details because they were negative.

Be Careful When Using Template Charts

Template (check-off) charting is useful for billing documentation. It is also frequently helpful in reminding us of important issues. However, there are several potential problems.

First, be sure to actually do everything you indicate that you did. Sometimes it is tempting to check off items that were not actually performed. Second, place your checkmarks carefully. Be sure your marks are in the correct squares. Finally, always write or dictate a summary note, except in the most routine cases (e.g., ankle sprain or sore throat). It is very difficult to defend your thought process if it is not apparent from the chart. Check marks and circles do not explain why you sent that chest pain patient home.

Read the Nursing Notes

Read these notes—even if they are not written for you. (The same rule applies to for paramedic notes.) Physicians often feel that the nursing notes are not relevant to them. This may sometimes be true for inpatient charting, such as noting family visits, bowel movements, and so on.

However, ED nursing notes are rarely irrelevant. Still, many physicians do not read them. I have seen many legal cases lost and a few won because of the nursing notes. You should read them before entering the examining room, periodically during the course of the patient's stay, and certainly when you write or dictate your own notes.

If you disagree with something in the nursing notes, then mention that in your own notes and the reason that you feel the nursing note is not correct. Never leave a clinically significant discrepancy unmentioned. The same principles apply to paramedic notes.

Nurses and paramedics often function under severe time constraints and may not complete their charting until much later. Three rules you should follow in reviewing nursing and paramedic notes include the following: (a) Beware of notes written after the patient leaves the emergency department; (b) beware of notes written after you have completed your chart; and (c) document if the paramedic notes are not available to you.

After-Care Instructions Are Crucial Both in Writing and in Reality

Ensure that your patient understands what to do. Studies have shown that as many as two-thirds of patients have no idea what the instructions they were given actually say. And most do not actually read the instructions anyway.

Review the after-care instructions with the patient yourself, at least verbally. Ideally, have the patient repeat the instructions back to you, preferably in a language you both understand. Use a translator if appropriate. Be sure to ask if the patient has any questions. You can then have the nurse provide written instructions and explain them one more time when the patient is actually discharged.

Be sure written instructions are in plain English (or Spanish, etc.) Many excellent computerized after-care instructions are available, often with a choice of various languages. Avoid medical terms and abbreviations such as "return prn."

If timely follow-up with another physician is crucial, then try to phone that physician to ensure that the patient can be seen expeditiously, and, of course, document the conversation.

I would strongly urge that family be included in the instruction process. Often, the patient is too distracted by pain, fear, or relief to fully comprehend your instructions. If there is any question of altered level of consciousness, such as head injury, then instructing the family is particularly crucial.

Be Sure to Follow Up Delayed Lab or X-Ray Reports

The ED is particularly vulnerable in following up lab or X-ray reports. The final results of many of the studies you order are not available to you before the patient is discharged. Culture and radiology reports are always delayed.

Every physician has been handed a urine culture or X-ray report that requires him or her to contact a patient seen by a colleague 1 or 2 days previously. The physician then asks a secretary to phone the patient, perhaps after he or she has gotten a busy signal. And often the physician forgets about the entire situation.

Sometimes, the phone number is absent or incorrect, in which case a letter should be sent and a copy added to the patient's chart. A certified letter is recommended. Occasionally, it may be appropriate to ask the police to go to the patient's residence.

This is an area of extreme liability for emergency physicians. Make sure your department has a formal protocol for follow-up of delayed reports. Make sure the follow-up process is completed. And of course, document! Your actions should become a part of the patient's permanent medical record.

Beware of Change-of-Shift

It is often necessary to transfer care of our patients to a newly arrived colleague at shift change. Both physicians are potentially liable for the patient's care. If you are the transferring physician, make sure your colleague has all the necessary information both verbally and, if appropriate, in writing. Remember that hours later, he or she may not remember everything you say, and your dictated report will usually not be available to your colleague.

If you are the receiving physician, make no assumptions. Do your own brief exam of the relevant systems. Review all study results. Re-evaluate if conditions change. Be sure that you are comfortable with the situation before discharge. Remember that responsibility for the patient has been transferred to you.

Temporary Admission (Holding) Orders

Many emergency physicians feel uncomfortable writing temporary admission orders. Others do not mind. Sometimes it depends on the situation. The official policy statement of the American College of Emergency Physicians (ACEP) states that emergency physicians should not be compelled to write such orders and should do so only when they feel comfortable. You do bear some responsibility for the patient so long as your orders are in effect and until the admitting physician has seen the patient.

Although this is an area of potential liability, temporary admission orders may be appropriate, and can be done in a manner that minimizes liability to you and danger to the patient. However, several things must be ensured and must be clearly understood by all parties involved:

1. Who is in charge of the patient?
2. Who knows it?
3. What is the life span of the data?
4. What is the life span of the orders?

Communication is crucial—between you and the floor nurses, between you and the admitting physician, and between the floor nurses and the admitting physician. Make sure there is no confusion. Orders should clearly specify (a) which doctor is responsible for the patient after admission and (b) whom to call, when to call, and for what reasons. For example, these orders might be necessary if questions or problems or breach of vital sign limits occur, or if the patient has not been seen by a specified time.

The temporary holding orders are necessarily based on data that has a life span and you won't be around if the data change. For example, make sure your fluid orders are time- or volume-limited. Specify what signs or symptoms the nurses should check (e.g., periodic neurological assessment of head injury patients or circulation checks for limb injuries).

An example of temporary admitting orders might include the following:

- Admit to Dr. X.
- Call Dr. X if questions or problems, or if Dr. X has not seen the patient by 6 PM.
- Vital signs every 2 hours.
- Call Dr. X if pulse less than 60 or greater than 100, or if blood pressure less than 110 systolic or 60 diastolic.

Emergency Medical Treatment and Active Labor Act

The federal Emergency Medical Treatment and Active Labor Act (EMTALA) is the official name for the law governing the transfer or discharge of patients from EDs. It is sometimes referred to by the aptly abbreviated acronym COBRA, a reference to the original Congressional legislation of which it was a section (the Consolidated Omnibus Budget Reconciliation Act of 1986).

Several important aspects of EMTALA must be stressed. First, a medical screening examination must be performed prior to inquiring about financial matters. However, this does not have to be performed by a physician, although that is the practice in many EDs. If a nurse performs the initial screening exam, he or she should be certified by the hospital to do so in accordance with a formal hospital protocol.

Second, the patient must be stabilized prior to transfer using the hospital's capabilities and must not be in active labor. Unfortunately, despite periodic federal guideline revisions, the word *stabilization* has never been clearly defined. And different regional jurisdictions have ruled differently on this matter.

Third, active labor means that the patient is likely to deliver prior to arrival at the receiving hospital.

Fourth, EMTALA governs discharge from the ED, regardless of destination. This includes discharge to home.

Fifth, patients may be transferred even if unstable, if they are transferred for medical reasons to a higher level of care facility. This might include cardiac patients transferred for catheterization or trauma patients sent to a trauma center. However, prior to transfer, the patient must be stabilized as much as possible.

Sixth, emergency physicians may be exempt from liability if forced to transfer an unstable patient. Thanks to the efforts of the ACEP, EMTALA excuses emergency physicians forced to transfer unstable patients because they cannot obtain an appropriate admitting physician or because the hospital refuses to admit the patient. However, the emergency physician must clearly state the reason and should identify the specialty physician who refused the admission, especially if that physician is formally on call to the ED. In such cases, however, the emergency physician must do what he or she can to stabilize the patient, such as starting intravenous fluids and antibiotics in a severely dehydrated, septic child or relieving the tension pneumothorax in a trauma patient.

Seventh, a bad result is not required for an EMTALA violation. The patient may have suffered no harm, yet an EMTALA violation may have occurred.

Eighth, EMTALA does not preclude transfer, even for economic reasons. Patients can be transferred from a private to a county hospital if they have no insurance or from a hospital that does not contract with their insurer to one that does. However, EMTALA does require that the patient be stabilized first. Unfortunately, the definition of the word *stabilization* is not always clear. However, as in all issues discussed in this chapter, the best practice is to do the right thing. Good medical care is the best defense against liability.

SPECIFIC MEDICAL CONDITIONS

The topics in this section represent a few of the most common entities resulting in lawsuits against emergency physicians and other doctors who treat patients in the ED. Obviously, this discussion is not meant to be a treatise on these topics but rather a reminder to be aware of some aspects of these conditions that are liable to be overlooked and result in litigation.

Chest Pain

Acute myocardial infarction (AMI) may require serial electrocardiograms and serum markers for diagnosis. Results may be non-diagnostic in the early hours of AMI. If pain suspicious for cardiac ischemia continues or recurs while in the ED, then studies should be repeated, often frequently.

Acute angina may quickly become lethal. When ST segments or cardiac markers are elevated, diagnosis of AMI is easy. However, when they are normal, beware of unstable angina. It may not be an infarct yet, but it may be lethal. Just because the pain has stopped does not mean the patient can be discharged to follow up in several days with a primary care physician. If there is any significant possibility of unstable angina, then arrange for admission and further treatment, or at least consult a cardiologist.

Pleuritic chest pain can be cardiac. The heart sits on the diaphragm. It moves with respiration. Cardiac ischemia thus can be pleuritic. The crucial question to distinguish pleural etiology from others causes is: Does it hurt between breaths? Pleural pain generally does not. Pleuritic cardiac pain may be worse with breathing, but it will definitely hurt between breaths as well.

Aortic dissection is more lethal than AMI. If the cardiac workup is negative even without back pain, then think about aortic dissection.

Pulmonary embolus may be accompanied by relatively normal oxygenation. Do not dismiss normal oxygen saturation, particularly if the respiratory rate is elevated.

When you discharge chest pain patients, let them and their family know that you cannot absolutely rule out cardiac or other serious etiology at that point in time. Document the discussion.

Abdominal Pain Can Always Be Appendicitis or Anything Else

Serious abdominal disorders often take time to develop. For many patients, more than one physician or ED visit is necessary for final diagnosis of appendicitis. When you discharge patients, let them and their family know that you cannot absolutely rule out appendicitis or other serious disorders at that point in time. Document the discussion.

Ischemic bowel is not very common and may not be considered. If subjective pain is out of proportion to a relatively non-tender abdomen on palpitation, think of this entity in older patients. Positive findings often include guaiac positive stools and metabolic acidosis.

Ruptured abdominal aortic aneurysm may present like renal colic, with left flank pain and even hematuria. Consider this possibility, particularly in older men.

Headache: Migraine, Tension, Drug Hit, or Subarachnoid Hemorrhage?

Most headaches are benign. However, subarachnoid hemorrhage (SAH) should be suspected if there is a sudden onset of pain, maximizing in 1–2 minutes and/or it is "the worst headache" of one's life.

Computed tomography (CT) scan may miss 2–10% of SAHs, depending on the scanner. If the above history is obtained and the CT scan is negative, then lumbar puncture is mandatory.

Clearing the Cervical Spine Includes Clearing the Cord as Well as the Bones

Remember SCIWORA (spinal cord injury without radiologic abnormality). Neurological dysfunction does not show up on film. Neurological symptoms or abnormalities on exam, despite a negative cervical spine X-ray, require further evaluation.

Medical Clearance for Psychiatry Patients

The goal is to differentiate organic from nonorganic etiology. This is done by evaluating cognition on the mental status exam.

To assess cognitive function, assess the level of consciousness, orientation, memory, attention, and fund of information.

No matter how psychotic he or she may seem, a schizophrenic or a person with a mood (affective) disorder, either bipolar or unipolar, will have normal cognition. Patients with altered levels of consciousness from toxic, metabolic, structural, or other nonpsychiatric causes will have altered cognition.

Be aware that no one can truly be medically cleared in the ED. They can be judged medically nonemergent at a given point in time. Document the clearance as such.

Chronically demented elderly patients deteriorate gradually. Do not assume an acute deterioration to be merely worsening of underlying Alzheimer's dementia. Any abrupt change in mental status in such patients often results from infection or medication.

Serious Knee Injury May Not Be Obvious

Ligament damage may be obscured by pain, effusion, or muscle spasm. Serious vascular injury may not impair circulation initially.

Popliteal artery contusion from transient knee dislocation may be associated with normal pulses at first but may result in delayed thrombosis and loss of limb. All knee dislocations require an arteriogram. Be careful not to confuse a history of an apparent patellar dislocation with a true knee joint dislocation.

Cauda Equina Syndrome

Do not forget to inquire about the status of the autonomic system in all patients with back pain. Ask about bowel and bladder function, both incontinence and incomplete evacuation. Impairment of urination or defecation is an ominous sign and requires immediate neurosurgical evaluation, usually including STAT magentic resonance imaging (MRI).

Epidural Abscess

Epidural abscess may be catastrophic yet quite inapparent. The patient typically presents with back pain, often thoracic, but with minimal findings on exam of either musculoskeletal or neurologic impairment.

Repeat visits to the ED for back pain should raise your suspicion of this disorder. Epidural abscess is a special danger in illicit needle users, precisely the population who may be faking or exaggerating illness to obtain narcotics. Thus, you should be very cautious in dismissing a complaint of severe back pain in needle users. If there is a possibility of epidural abscess, an MRI is usually diagnostic.

Endotracheal Intubation

Inadvertent esophageal intubation may result in good breath sounds. This is particularly common in small children with uncuffed tubes. Even if you place the tube correctly, it can become dislodged as the patient is moved or manipulated for X-rays.

At least several of the following methods should be used to confirm correct tube position. (Be sure to document.)

- Symmetric breath sounds.
- Absence of gastric sounds.
- Vapor in the tube with each breath.
- Good compliance with bagging.
- Increased, and hopefully adequate, oxygen saturation.
- Carbon dioxide detector variation with each breath.

- Spontaneous insufflation between breaths, of a large compressible bulb attached to a correctly placed endotracheal tube. Lack of spontaneous insufflation indicates esophageal placement.

Be sure the tube is secured correctly, even if performed by a respiratory therapist.

Drug Addicts May Also Be Sick

Drug-seeking behavior, with false claims of illness, is common in EDs. However, drug abusers, especially illicit needle users, are more prone to true illness than the general population. Consider needle users to be immunosuppressed. Beware of occult infection, especially epidural abscess. Illicit drug users frequently exhibit tachyphylaxis to narcotic analgesics. If they need pain medication, they usually need more than nonaddicts.

Do Not Lose Your Patient in X-Ray

One last thing to remember: it is easy to forget patients sent out of the ED for studies. Use of a tracking board may help. If the patient is unstable, then send a nurse.

CONCLUSION

Malpractice litigation and the fear of being sued are unfortunate aspects of practicing medicine in American culture. As Bob Dylan once opined, "Everybody must get stoned." However, we can definitely minimize that risk by practicing good medicine and by communicating with our patients in an open and caring manner. Never forget the importance of good documentation in the medical record.

It is often said that physicians have already lost just by being sued, even if they ultimately win the case. It is an agonizing experience to be called a bad doctor when you know that you did not commit malpractice. And if you think that you really did do something suboptimal, then you have to deal with your own guilt.

I would strongly suggest availing yourself of professional counseling if depression, guilt, or anger are significant. Many local and state medical associations have support groups for doctors involved in malpractice litigation. It is important to realize that no matter what happens in the legal case in question, it is an aberration. Physicians treat thousands of patients in their careers, and far more than 99% of patients are helped by their physicians' care.

In the end, the best defense against being sued is to practice good medicine. As has been mentioned previously: do the right thing. If you are a good doctor, communicate well with your patients, and pay attention to documentation, you will have gone a long way toward not only preventing lawsuits but also truly helping the people who come to you for care.

SUGGESTED READINGS

1. Schumacher JE, Ritchey FJ, Nelson LT 3rd. Malpractice litigation fear and risk management beliefs among teaching hospital physicians. South Med J 1995; 88(12):1204.
2. Ransom SB, Dombrowski MP, Shephard R, Leonardi M. The economic cost of the medical-legal tort system. Am J Obstet Gynecol 1996;174(6):1903.
3. Brennan TA, Sox CM, Burstin HR. Relation between negligent adverse events and the outcomes of medical malpractice litigation. N Engl J Med 1966;33(26): 1963.
4. Bovbjerg RR, Petronis KR. The relationship between physicians' malpractice claims history and later claims: does the past predict the future? JAMA 1994;272(18): 1421.
5. Posner KL, Caplan RA, Cheney FW. Variation in expert opinion in medical malpractice review. Anesthesiology 1996;85(5):1049.
6. Hyams AL, Brandenburg JA, Lipsitz SR, Shapiro DW, Brennan TA. Practice guidelines and malpractice litigation: a two-way street. Ann Intern Med 1995; 122(6):450.
7. American College of Emergency Physicians Clinical Policies. Website: accep.org.
8. Karcz A, Holbrook J, Auerbach BS, et al. Preventability of malpractice claims in emergency medicine: A closed claims study. Ann Emerg Med 1990;19(8):865.
9. Johnson LA, Derlet RW. Conflicts between managed care organizations and emergency departments in California. West J Med 1996;164(2):137.
10. Derlet RW, Hamilton B. The impact of health maintenance organization care authorization policy on an emergency department before California's new managed care law. Acad Emerg Med 1996;3(4):338.
11. Lerman B, Kobernick MS. Return visits to the emergency department. J Emerg Med 1987;5(5):359.
12. Hirsch H. Legal implications of patient records. South Med J 1979;72(6):726.
13. Prosser RL Jr. Alteration of medical records submitted for medicolegal review. JAMA 1992;276(19):2630.
14. Powers RD. Emergency department patient literacy and the readability of patient-directed materials. Ann Emerg Med 1988;17(2):124.
15. Simel DL, Feussner JR. Does determining serum alcohol concentrations in emergency department patients influence physicians' civil suit liability? Arch intern Med 1989;149(5)1016.
16. Martin CA, Wilson JF, Fiebelman ND 3rd, Gurley DN, Miller TW. Physicians' psychologic reactions to malpractice litigation. South Med J. 1991; 84(11):1300.
17. Lester GW, Smith SG. Listening and talking to patients: a remedy for malpractice suits? West J Med 1993;158(3):268.

10 Anesthesiology

Ann S. Lofsky, MD

SUMMARY

This chapter reviews the leading causes for anesthesiology malpractice claims and the indemnity payments that result from different patient injuries. Risk-management strategies are provided
both to help prevent patient injuries and to make anesthesia
claims more defensible. The effect of anesthesia claims on the
physician is discussed.

Key Words: Anesthesiology; American Society of Anesthesiologists (ASA) monitoring standards; frequency; severity; claims
trends; informed consent.

INTRODUCTION

In the 20 years since the widespread adoption of new monitoring
technologies in anesthesia, the specialty has gone from high to low risk
in the rating systems of most malpractice carriers. It is often cited as a
role model for specialties seeking to improve patient outcomes and
decrease the likelihood of malpractice litigation. Anesthesiology currently has one of the lowest incidences of claim frequency among all
specialties, with anesthesiologists sued an average of once every 8
years. The nature of the claims themselves has also changed with a
marked decline in the percentages of claims for catastrophic injures

From: *Medical Malpractice: A Physician's Sourcebook*
Edited by: R. E. Anderson © Humana Press Inc., Totowa, NJ

such as brain damage and death. As a result, in inflation-adjusted dollars, anesthesia is one of the few specialties to see declining premiums.

This decrease in catastrophic cases is largely attributable to the monitoring capabilities supplied by the pulse oximeter and end-tidal carbon dioxide (CO_2) monitors. These came into widespread use in the 1990s and are now included in American Society of Anesthesiologists (ASA) monitoring standards. These monitors, when used correctly, have virtually eliminated unrecognized esophageal intubations in the operating room and serve as an early warning sign of inadequate ventilation, something that only 15 years ago, surgeons first recognized by noticing darker blood in the surgical site.

The practice of anesthesiology itself has undergone radical changes in recent years. General anesthesia now includes options of both inhalational (gas) anesthetics and total intravenous agents. Difficult intubations are aided by newer visualization techniques or eliminated by the use of the laryngeal mask airway (LMA). Many cases can now be performed with monitored anesthesia care (MAC; intravenous sedation) or regional neurological block techniques. These newer alternatives have improved patient safety by allowing anesthetics to be specifically tailored to the patient's needs and physical limitations.

Many anesthesiologists now work outside the operating room in intensive care units or as pain specialists in freestanding office practices. By working in these areas, anesthesiologists have overlapped the traditional practices of family practitioners, physical medicine physicians, and neurologists, among others. Malpractice insurance companies have had to struggle to assess and appropriately price these new risks and to decide whether these anesthesiologists rightly belong to separate specialties, such as pain or intensive medicine. The discussion of pain and other nontraditional anesthesiology practices is beyond the scope of this chapter, which is intended to focus on claims related to operating room, surgery center, office operating room, and obstetrical anesthesia.

CLAIMS

To study anesthesia claim trends, The Doctors Company (TDC), a national physician-owned medical malpractice insurance company, looked at a representative sample of 500 consecutive anesthesia claims. Of the 500 claims, 456 had closed at the time of the review. Of the closed claims, 51 (11%) resulted in indemnity payments. Malpractice indemnity, by definition, is a dollar payout on behalf of the phy-

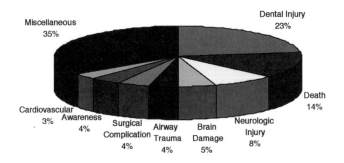

Fig.1. Anesthesia claims by injury.

sician either as a result of a settlement or adverse jury verdict. Correspondingly, 89% of these anesthesia claims closed without any payment being made to the plaintiff, which is a better defense rate than observed for many other specialties. Overall, TDC closes approx 80% of claims without indemnity payments.

Figure 1 shows the distribution of the 500 claims by injury. Dental damage is the single most common allegation in anesthesia claims, accounting for nearly one-fourth of the claims studied here. About half of these are a result of trauma during endotracheal intubation, with the other half involving patients biting down on hard objects such as plastic oral airways and LMA shafts—often in the recovery period. The most commonly injured teeth in these claims are the upper front incisors, with injuries to prosthetic dental work such as crowns and bridges as another common allegation.

Claims involving a patient death in the perioperative period occur in 14% of the claims in this series. Many of these claims do not involve obvious anesthesia errors; however, frequently in malpractice cases involving a death, numerous physicians are named initially and later dropped after discovery proceeds. Only 8% of the death claims resulted in indemnity payments. However, those cases that did pay indemnity had an average payout of $225,000 to the decedent's family.

Malpractice claims alleging neurological injuries are almost evenly divided between general anesthetics, in which improper positioning may be an issue, and epidural and spinal block cases, in which direct nerve trauma can occur. Brain damage claims comprise 5% of claims in this series and include cases of severe anoxic injury resulting from loss of the airway and respiratory insufficiency. This category includes some of the most expensive claims in this series. Airway trauma claims, comprising 4% of the claims reviewed here, include pharyngeal tears and esophageal perforations—usually resulting from difficult endotracheal intubation attempts. Only 1 of the 20 airway trauma cases here paid indemnity, although TDC paid $90,000 on that single case. Airway trauma can be considered within the risks of normal anesthesia care, as endotracheal intubation may be required in difficult circumstances for the anesthesiologist. This likely explains the low percentage of indemnity payouts for this type of claim.

Lawsuits listed as surgical complications include cases where, based on the allegation, a peer reviewer felt there was minimal probability of an anesthesia contribution, but the anesthesiologist was named largely because of a poor surgical outcome. An example of this type of case would be a claim involving an accidental ligation of the common bile duct during laparoscopic cholecystectomy, in which the anesthesiologist was named along with the primary and assistant surgeons. Of the 20 cases considered to have resulted from surgical complications, only 1 paid an indemnity to the patient. This was a settlement for $10,000, considered nominal by medical malpractice standards.

Although they frequently receive considerable attention in the media, malpractice claims alleging unanticipated awareness under anesthesia comprise only about 4% of claims seen here. Interestingly, not all of these cases involved recall under general anesthesia. Approximately one-third of the claims involved regional blocks or intravenous sedation anesthetics with intentionally awake patients; in these cases, patient expectation and informed consent become issues. Clearly, patients who understand and accept in advance that they are expected to be awake, but pain-free, for a portion or all of their surgical procedures are less likely to sue when this occurs. The total indemnity paid on awareness claims was $15,000, indicating that this is not a major malpractice issue.

Cardiovascular injuries account for 3% of these claims. These cases involve plaintiffs who suffered strokes or myocardial infarctions in the perioperative period and who allege that anesthesia may have been a contributing factor. The large miscellaneous group includes less frequently named patient injuries, which (listed in decreasing frequency) are neurologically impaired infant claims (alleging that maternal anesthesia was a factor), operations on the incorrect surgical site, painful anesthesia, aspiration pneumonia, falls off the operating room table, postspinal headache, and medication errors.

Figure 2 shows the total indemnity dollars for each category of paid anesthesia claims. The chart shows the top eight injury payouts, in

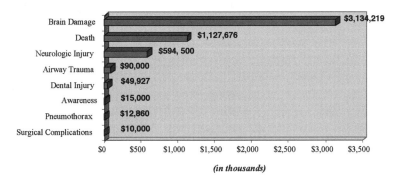

$5,034,182

Fig. 2. Indemnity payments.

order, as brain damage, death, neurological injury, airway trauma, dental injury, awareness, pneumothorax, and surgical complication. Although dental injury is by far the most common allegation in anesthesia claims, it certainly is not the most expensive in terms of indemnity dollars paid, accounting for only 1% of the $5 million total. The most expensive injuries, as might be expected, are the most severe. Brain damage and death account for 62 and 22%, respectively, of the total dollars paid. Brain damage, proportionally, is the single most expensive injury, accounting for only 5% of the claims by number but nearly two-thirds of the dollars paid on behalf of anesthesiologists. This is largely explained by the requirement of many of these injured plaintiffs for lifetime medical care and for reimbursement of lifetime loss of income.

The indemnity for brain damage cases averaged $630,000 per claim paid, which is the highest average for any injury in this series. Death cases, as stated previously, averaged $225,000 in indemnity per case. For neurological injuries paying indemnity, the average per claim was $119,000. Dental injures, by comparison, averaged only $1700 per claim; this, of course, does not reflect the administrative costs incurred by the insurance company in handling the relatively large number of dental claims.

Figure 3 shows the percentage of claims for each injury for which indemnity was paid. Dental injury has the highest percentage of claims paid, with indemnity paid on 30 out of 103 (29%) claims. Brain damage claims have the second highest percentage of indemnity payouts,

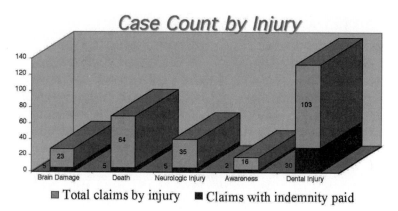

Case Count by Injury

■ Total claims by injury   ■ Claims with indemnity paid

Fig. 3. Number of claims closed with indemnity paid.

with dollars paid to close 22% of those claims. Next highest in frequency are neurological injuries, of which 14% were closed with indemnity. Awareness claims had a similar percentage, with 13% making payments to plaintiffs. Only 8% of claims involving patient death closed with indemnity paid on behalf of the anesthesiologist.

RISK MANAGEMENT: IMPROVING PATIENT AND LEGAL OUTCOMES

Risk management has long been a concern for TDC, with aims to both prevent patient injury and increase the defensibility of negative outcomes that are considered to be within the risks of the specialty. Risk-management publications for anesthesiology have largely been driven by perceived claims trends and typically follow peer-group discussions of representative claims.

Documentation

One of the factors involved in deciding to take an anesthesiology claim to trial is the quality of the charting. The anesthesia record, preoperative sheet, and informed consent are legal documents that like other medical records, are admissible in court. In a malpractice trial involving an anesthesiology issue, typically the anesthesia records will be projected on a screen or enlarged to poster-size to be placed in front of a jury. The anesthesiologist might then be asked to interpret or explain what has been recorded. Illegible or incomplete records can be a major problem at trial, because plaintiff attorneys may use missing or unclear information to imply that the anesthesiologist might have been sloppy in the care of the patient, not merely in the recording of it. Anesthesiologists are strongly encouraged to write legibly and to make sure that entries are correctly timed and as accurate as possible. Notes that are written out of sequence or added late to a record should be clearly labeled as such. A number of anesthesia claims have been settled when it was determined that portions of the medical record were altered after the fact, apparently in a misguided effort to render the claims more defensible.

Record keeping is particularly important when untoward events occur. Often, an anesthesiologist's attention is correctly directed toward caring for the patient, not on charting. If something out of the ordinary occurs, such as an arrest or anaphylactic reaction, then it is suggested that once the situation has resolved, the anesthesiologist write a separate narrative in the medical record detailing the sequence of events and the treatment rendered. Often, standard anesthesia forms have minimal space provided for written descriptions, and this may not be sufficient for the kind of detail that would later be useful in defending the medical care provided.

Charting in advance can be a problem. Although anesthesiologists sometimes fill out portions of the record in advance to save time on routine cases, they run the risk that subsequent events might not correspond to what has already been charted. From a legal standpoint, this could make it appear that the entire record is fraudulent *(1)*.

Informed Consent

Anesthesia claims, like claims for other specialties, can hinge on issues of informed consent. Particularly when there are alternative methods a patient could have chosen (i.e., general, regional, MAC), plaintiffs might allege they would have chosen differently and avoided complications had they been given the choice. Personal recall is unreliable, and the written record of the informed consent process is usually the most persuasive evidence in court. The old risk-management adage, "If you didn't write it down, it didn't happen," seems unfair but often holds true in litigation. Sometimes, anesthesia records include minimal or no documentation of the informed consent, rendering otherwise defensible claims more problematic.

Good documentation of the informed consent need not be extensive. Often, this includes a simple summary of the risks discussed, for example: "Risks of general anesthesia explained, including possible sore throat, dental injury, pneumonia, and death." Patients can be reassured that although the risks mentioned are highly unlikely, they have been known to occur and they should be aware that nothing in life, including anesthesia, is risk-free.

Informed consent can be difficult on labor and delivery, where a patient might first be met when she is in active labor, but it is certainly no less important in this situation. Claims resulting from epidural or spinal anesthetics on pregnant patients often include allegations of back pain or postspinal headaches that are considered within the risks of the procedure. Documenting that this was explained in advance can go a long way toward making these claims defensible. An example of informed consent for an epidural anesthetic would be: "Infrequently patients get headaches from placement of the epidural. If you do get a headache, there are treatments available. Other uncommon complications are backache, nerve injury, or even death" (1).

Some anesthesiologists feel more comfortable using preprinted informed consent forms or checklists listing the procedures and risks discussed. From a malpractice company's perspective, anything documenting this process can go a long way toward eliminating an informed consent issue from a claim. TDC has developed an informed consent form at the request of insureds that can be used, if desired, in lieu of a handwritten informed consent. It is printed as a double-sided form and is signed by both the patient and the anesthesia provider. A copy is provided in Fig. 4.

INJURY PREVENTION

In addition to generalized risk-management suggestions, which help make all claims more defensible, recommendations may be made regarding practice patterns that might help prevent specific patient injuries from occurring or help prevent those injuries from triggering claims. Usually, these recommendations are derived from claim reviews and peer-member review panels looking at groups of claims where plaintiffs have alleged similar injuries.

Dental Injury

Injuries to natural teeth and prosthetic dental work are by far the most common reasons anesthesiologists are sued. Although usually these cases are settled for relatively small amounts of money, there is still the stress of being sued on the physician and concerns about reporting requirements to the National Practitioner Data Bank. Currently, any settlement or indemnity payment made on behalf of a physician must be reported to this centralized reporting agency, regardless

ANESTHESIA

Anesthesia is a specialty medical service which administers anesthetic agents to, and manages patients who are rendered unconscious or diminished response to pain and stress during the course of a medical, surgical, or obstetrical procedure.

TYPES OF ANESTHESIA AND DEFINITIONS

A. **General Anesthesia**
1. Endotracheal anesthesia *Anesthetic and respiratory gases are passed through a tube placed in the trachea (windpipe) via the nose or mouth.*
2. Mask anesthesia *Gases are passed through a mask which covers the nose and mouth.*
3. Laryngeal mask airway (LMA) *Gases are passed through the endotracheal tube that is attached to a small mask, though the tube does not pass through the vocal cords.*

B. **Regional Anesthesia**
1. Epidural anesthesia *A small catheter is inserted into epidural (spinal) space so that anesthetizing agents may be given to prolong the duration of anesthesia.*
2. Spinal anesthesia *The anesthetic agent is injected into the spinal subarachnoid space to produce loss of sensation.*
3. Nerve blocks *Local anesthetizing agents are injected into specific areas to inhibit nerve transmission.*

C. **Monitored Anesthesia Care (MAC):** *includes the monitoring of at least blood pressure, oxygenation, pulse and mental state, supplementing sedation and analgesia as needed.*

D. **Sedation**
1. Conscious Sedation *is a medically controlled state of depressed consciousness that: 1) allows protective reflexes to be maintained; 2) retains the patient's ability to maintain a patent airway independently and continuously, and 3) permits appropriate response by the patient to verbal command.*
2. Deep Sedation *is a medically controlled state of depressed consciousness or unconsciousness from which the patient is not easily aroused, which may be accompanied by a partial or complete loss of reflexes, including the ability to patent airway independently and respond purposefully to verbal command.*

E. **Local Anesthesia**
1. Local anesthesia *Anesthetizing agents are injected or infiltrated directly into a small area of the body, for example, the surgical site.*
2. Topical anesthesia *Surface anesthesia is produced by direct application of anesthetizing agents on skin or mucous membranes.*

Patient's
Initials

_____ The details of the procedure have been explained to me in terms I understand.

_____ Alternative methods and their benefits and disadvantages have been explained to me.

_____ I understand and accept the most likely risks and complications but are not limited to:

allergic/adverse reaction	*nausea*
aspiration	*ophthalmic (eye) injury*
backache	*pain*
brain damage	*paralysis*
coma	*pneumonia*
dental damage	*positional nerve injury*
headache	*recall of sound/noise/speech by others*
inability to reverse the effects of anesthesia	*seizure*
infection	*sore throat*
localized swelling and or redness	*wrong site for injection of anesthesia*
muscle aches	

continued

7/00

Fig. 4. Anesthesia informed consent form (Copyright © The Doctors Company).

of the monetary amount. From a malpractice carrier's standpoint, there are defense costs related to the handling of this relatively large volume of claims. Although a patient may be complaining of a single broken tooth, the handling of that claim might require an interview with the insured, letters to the plaintiff, reports from dentists, and subpoenas of hospital records.

_____ I understand that accidental dental injury is also a risk of anesthesia. The anesthesiologist cannot be held responsible for injuring teeth, partials, or dentures that are already damaged or in poor condition.

_____ I understand and accept the less common complications, including the remote risk of death or serious disability that exists with any anesthesia procedure.

_____ I am aware that smoking during the pre- and postoperative periods could increase chances of complications.

_____ I have informed the doctor of all my known allergies.

_____ I have informed the doctor of all medications I am currently taking, including prescriptions, over-the-counter remedies, herbal therapies, and any other.

_____ I have been advised whether I should avoid taking any or all of these medications on the days surrounding the procedure date.

_____ I am aware and accept that no guarantees about the results of the procedure have been made.

_____ The doctor has answered all of my questions regarding this procedure.

I certify that I have read and understand this procedure agreement and that all blanks were filled in prior to my signature.

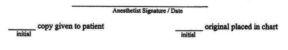

| Patient or Legal Representative Signature / Date | Relationship (self, parent, etc.) |

| Print Patient or Legal Representative Name | Witness Signature / Date |

I certify that I have explained the nature, purpose, benefits, risks, complications, and alternatives to the proposed procedure to the patient or the patient's legal representative. I have answered all questions fully, and I believe that the *patient / legal representative* (circle one) fully understands what I have explained.

| Anesthetist Signature / Date |

_____ copy given to patient   _____ original placed in chart
initial   initial

Fig. 4. *(Continued)*

Dental injury claims constitute 23% of all anesthesia claims but account for 59% of all cases paying indemnity. Although only 11% of anesthesia claims overall will pay indemnity, 29% of dental injury claims will ultimately result in payments. This high rate of payment is likely related to the clear causation link between the anesthetic and the broken or damaged teeth. Often, an anesthesiologist is aware at the time of surgery that teeth have been broken, or the patient may complain soon afterward in the recovery room or before leaving the hospital. The teeth most commonly injured during anesthesia are the two upper front incisors (numbers 8 and 9), which are vulnerable to laryngoscope pressure during visualization of the vocal cords and to pressure from a semi-awake patient biting down directly on a hard substance. These upper teeth may be bonded or capped for cosmetic reasons, making them even more vulnerable to damage. Prosthetic dental work, like permanent bridges, also seem particularly vulnerable to problems during airway management.

Anesthesiologists are encouraged to specifically inquire about pre-existing dental work, especially in the front of the mouth. If invasive airway management (such as endotracheal tube or LMA placement) is planned, anything that is usually removable by the patient should be taken out of the mouth in advance. Anesthesiologists are also encouraged to specifically examine their patients' teeth preoperatively, making written notations regarding pre-existing damage, especially to the front teeth. Chipped, broken, or loose teeth can be pointed out to the patient, who may not even be aware that such damage already exists. If vulnerable teeth are noted, the anesthesiologist can consider using plastic oral dental guards or gauze packs placed in the sides of the mouth to prevent voluntary occlusion. Oral airways can be removed or exchanged for nasal airways during recovery before a patient is awake enough to bite down forcibly.

Informed consents for general anesthesia should mention dental injury because it is so common and because patients who have been forewarned about this possibility are less likely to be angry and litigious should it actually occur. In the event of accidental dental injury, an anesthesiologist should be frank and honest with the patient about what has happened. In actuality, dental injury is within the risks of anesthesia, but anesthesiologists often become defensive, arguing, "It's not my fault, I didn't do anything wrong." Patients, on the other hand, often take the stance, "The tooth wasn't broken when I got here, and now it is, so you should pay me for it." This is the reason that insurance carriers typically must get involved.

Frequently, dental claims are settled by reimbursing the patient for the cost of repairing the teeth to their pre-anesthesia state. To avoid inflated estimates, an evaluation by an independent dentist, who will not actually be doing the repairs, is often sought. Anesthesiologists are advised to first try working with patients directly to get these situations resolved in a way that seems fair and equitable to everyone. Occasionally a dental claim does escalate, with the patient and anesthesiologist generating legal bills many times greater than the cost of the actual dental repairs. Any physician who reimburses a patient directly is advised to obtain a liability release from that patient accepting that as payment in full *(2)*.

Anesthesia Disasters

If dental injury is considered to be one end of a spectrum—a common, but minor, and sometimes unavoidable patient injury—the cases considered anesthetic disasters would comprise the spectrum's other end. These are cases in which anesthesia errors directly cause serious patient injuries, including brain damage or death. By definition, these cases could have been avoided. In an era of sophisticated anesthetic techniques and monitoring, it is easy to forget that cases like these still can and do occur. Peer review of these claims has led to a series of risk management suggestions.

MONITORING

Since the widespread adoption of the pulse oximeter and end-tidal CO_2 monitors, anesthesia has become much safer. However, serious injuries still result because of failures to use the monitors correctly. Inactivation of the pulse oximeter alarm accounts for a large proportion of anoxic injury cases that involve respiratory insufficiency that is noticed too late. Anoxic damage can occur within minutes of an unrecognized and untreated respiratory arrest, even in an operating room. Anesthesiologists should be very careful when silencing the auditory alarms on these monitors, especially if they are not positive they will remain directly in their line of sight. It is also important to remain vigilant with sedated patients having MAC or regional blocks, as the level of sedation can often deepen without warning. The scenario of an anesthesiologist who silenced a pulse oximeter alarm because of "false alarms" and then left the head of the bed or became otherwise distracted is seen in a very large proportion of these claims.

ESOPHAGEAL INTUBATION

Malpractice cases alleging esophageal intubation by the anesthesiologist still occur. Intubating the esophagus is not negligent, but the failure to promptly recognize the situation and replace the tube is. In many cases ultimately considered to involve unrecognized esophageal intubations, the anesthesiologists claimed they were sure the endotracheal tubes were correctly placed because they had watched them pass directly through the vocal cords. Alternatively, several argued that they had verified bilateral breath sounds over their patients' chests. In this day and age, for operating room anesthesia, an end-tidal CO_2 reading is the only acceptable method of proving correct endotrachial tube placement. Failure to immediately check and record an end-tidal CO_2 reading in the presence of a functioning CO_2 monitor would not likely be found to meet the standard of care.

Anesthesiologists sometimes simply fail to consider the possibility of an esophageal intubation when encountering problems immediately after intubating a patient. It is not uncommon to have anesthesiologists claim that they were sure they were dealing with bronchospasm or problems with the monitors before other physicians arrived to assist them, replacing the endotracheal tubes and correcting the problems. In a healthy preoxygenated patient, it may take up to 30 minutes before the blood pressure and heart rate become unstable in the event of an esophageal intubation. If any patient develops instability in this time frame, esophageal intubation should at least be considered and ruled out. If the anesthesiologist is unsure whether the tube is correctly placed, then it should be removed and the patient ventilated by other means, such as a facemask or LMA. An old adage regarding intubation states, "When in doubt, take it out!"

OBSTETRICS

Serious complications occur on labor and delivery wards as a direct result of anesthesia provided to patients for labor and obstetrical surgical procedures. An anesthesiologist in this situation often must confront concerns both for the mother and her baby. Decisions must be made in haste for the sake of a baby in peril, and a sense of urgency can pervade the anesthesia care as well. However, an anesthesiologist's primary responsibility is to the mother. Even emergency Cesarean sections (C-sections) can be delayed if there are concerns about the mother's safety. Several malpractice disasters have involved brain damage in the mother resulting from untreated respiratory arrest, because the anesthesiologist's attention was diverted in the hustle to transfer the patient for a crash C-section because the baby was unstable. Similarly, an anesthesiologist should not leave an unstable mother unattended to assist with her newborn.

Labor and delivery is a unique environment, where an anesthesiologist is often providing care to more than one parturient at a time. Anesthesia may be provided in the middle of the night, when there are few back-up personnel available. However, the standard of care otherwise varies little from similar procedures performed in the main operating room at any hour of the day. Care must be taken to ensure that the area is appropriately stocked with different airway equipment and emergency drugs and that labor and delivery staff are acquainted with the locations of these items.

Labor epidurals and spinals can take up to 30 minutes to develop their full effects, and someone, if not the anesthesiologist, should be checking the patient and her vital signs at intervals during this period.

Disasters have occurred when the anesthesiologist leaves a seemingly stable patient soon after placing a block to attend to another patient who appears to have a more urgent problem. When the second patient has been stabilized, it is suddenly realized that the first patient has suffered an unrecognized respiratory arrest because no one was in the room with her.

The physiologic changes of pregnancy may be partly responsible for the increased incidence of anoxic injuries during obstetrical care. Decreased pulmonary functional residual capacity in the mother greatly limits the duration of apnea required before serious hypoxia occurs. A healthy woman might survive a several-minute transfer time from the labor room to the surgical suite without ventilating. The same woman who is 9 months pregnant might not. A nonbreathing woman in labor is an emergency; nothing should be more important to an anesthesiologist than getting her ventilated and oxygenated. Babies in obstetrical cases seem possibly more resistant to periods of anoxia than mothers do. It is not unusual for disaster claims to involve an apparently healthy baby with normal Apgars who is born to a mother who developed severe anoxic brain damage from a predelivery apneic episode *(3)*.

OFFICE ANESTHESIA

Private office and surgery center operating rooms may provide environments that are quite different from what anesthesiologists are accustomed to in large hospital settings. Supplies and personnel might be relatively unfamiliar to anesthesiologists who do not practice at these sites frequently, but an emergency situation is never the optimal time to try to determine where needed drugs and equipment are stored. When practicing in situations new to them, anesthesiologists are advised to spend time in advance familiarizing themselves with the anesthesia equipment provided and learning where drugs and supplies are kept. This should include items such as emergency airway equipment and malignant hyperthermia supplies. Regardless of where anesthesiologists practice, they remain ultimately responsible for the safe conduct of anesthetics that they agree to perform. This includes the handling of any unforeseen complications that might develop within currently acceptable standards of care.

Anesthesiologists usually remain responsible for patients until they are stable in the recovery area and their care has been turned over to qualified personnel. Serious complications have occurred in office operating rooms when patients have been left after uneventful surgeries in recovery areas poorly designed for this function and with inadequate monitoring. Anesthesiologists should be aware of who will be watching their patients' vital signs and what monitors will be used. Postoperative orders that allow unfamiliar recovery personnel to make potentially crucial decisions regarding pain medication and discharge home might be handled quite differently than the same orders given in a hospital recovery room.

The changes in anesthesia practices needed to prevent most disaster cases are relatively minor and usually easily accomplished. Anesthesiologists should consider the times each day when their own patients could be vulnerable to disasters should circumstances conspire against them. These cases are devastating to patients, their loved ones, and often the physicians involved. No one wants to feel that they were involved in a claim that might have been easily preventable.

REGIONAL BLOCKS

Claims resulting from anesthesia provided by regional blocks, including epidural, spinal anesthetics, and brachial plexus blocks, often allege injuries different from claims involving general anesthesia. Panel reviews of these claims have found that the main allegations include nerve damage, inadequate volume replacement, informed consent, and patient communication problems.

Nerve damage injuries include allegations of pain, numbness, and palsies. However, not all nerve injuries are related to anesthesia. Often in obstetrical/gynecology claims, subsequent neurological consultation finds that the injuries are more consistent with saphenous or peroneal nerve damage from lithotomy stirrups or obturator nerve damage from compression against the pelvic bone during delivery. Still, a patient with weak or numb legs who has had an epidural is likely to assume that it is the cause. Similarly, when patients develop neurological symptoms after arm surgeries performed under brachial plexus blocks, it can be difficult to determine whether the cause is the surgery itself or the anesthetic. Therefore, anesthesiologists are advised to seek prompt neurological consultation for patients with persistent neurological complaints after regional blocks.

Anesthesiologists should always be cognizant of the risk of epidural hematoma formation after epidural blocks. Although this is a rare complication, cases and claims still do occur. Because the window for regaining function after cord compression from an epidural hematoma may be as small as 6–8 hours, often at issue in these claims is how promptly the hematoma was suspected and diagnosed, usually through magnetic resonance imaging scanning. Although plaintiffs often must concede that epidural hematomas are within the risks of the procedure, a failure to diagnose them in a reasonable time frame might not be. Because the risks of hematoma formation are higher when epidural catheters are used in combination with anticoagulants like heparin, warfarin, and enoxaparin (Lovenox®), anesthesiologists should communicate with surgeons and primary care physicians who could be writing anticoagulation orders for these drugs on their patients.

The issue of whether regional blocks should be placed in patients who are already under general anesthesia remains controversial. A number of claims have occurred related to placement of interscalene and supraclavicular brachial plexus blocks for postoperative pain relief in shoulder surgeries performed under general anesthesia. Injuries have included total arm paralysis and direct trauma to the spinal cord. In these cases, the blocks were placed after the patients were asleep. The allegation is always that if the patient had been awake when the block was performed, pain and paresthesias would have alerted the anesthesiologist to improper needle placement and avoided the severe neurological injury. Anesthesiologists should also carefully weigh the risks of performing thoracic and cervical epidural blocks on patients under general anesthesia or heavy sedation. These patients might not be completely cooperative or able to communicate uncomfortable sensations to their physicians.

Epidural and spinal blocks performed for surgical anesthesia often result in relative hypovolemia because of vasodilatation. Some anesthesia claims allege inappropriate use of these blocks in severely hypovolemic patients or inadequate replacement of the resulting intraoperative fluid shifts. Line placement may become an issue, because central venous catheters or Swan-Ganz catheter lines can help clarify patients' volume status if it is uncertain, although other factors such as blood pressure, heart rate, and urine output are also useful guides *(4)*.

Informed consent can become an issue in claims involving regional blocks simply because the alternative of general anesthesia usually exists. An anesthesiologist should provide some documentation that the more common risks of regional blockade were discussed with the patient and, ideally, that the alternatives to a block were also presented. If there are particular reasons why an anesthesiologist prefers a regional block, such as poor patient respiratory status or anticipated airway difficulties, then it is also helpful if this is recorded. Blocks performed solely for postoperative pain relief should be explained as such, and the alternatives should be presented to the patient.

Although considered well within the risks of epidural and spinal anesthetics, postsubdural puncture headaches remain a common cause of malpractice claims. As this is one of the more common complications, it should likely be mentioned in the informed consent for all planned epidurals and spinals. Should an accidental dural puncture occur in a planned epidural anesthetic or should a patient complain of a classic positional headache afterward, the anesthesiologist should evaluate the patient and explain alternatives to treatment, such as pain medication and blood patching. Many of these claims seem to arise when the patient has felt ignored or has had to endure a time-consuming and expensive process to be evaluated and treated by a physician for a headache complaint.

OPERATING ROOM FIRES

Historically, operating room fires were associated with flammable anesthetics and static electricity. Although flammable agents have largely disappeared from modern operating rooms, fires and the malpractice cases that can result from them unfortunately still remain. Modern developments such as electrical cautery, lasers, and paper and plastic disposables have enhanced the surgical environment while adding new risks of fire.

Three conditions must be present for a fire to occur in the operating room.

1. Fuel

    All materials can burn in an oxygen-enriched environment. These include drapes, dressings, gauze, surgical gowns, syringes, hair, gastrointestinal gases, petroleum-based ointments, and most plastics.

2. Oxidizer

    Both oxygen and nitrous oxide support fires. Any concentration of oxygen in excess of 21% should be considered enriched. These gases can accumulate around the operative site as well as under drapes and in body cavities, such as the oropharynx.

3. Ignition Source

    Heat sources typically include electrosurgical cautery, fiberoptic light sources, and lasers.

Any combination of an oxygen-enriched environment, a flammable material, and a heat source in the same place at the same time is an accident waiting to happen. It is not uncommon to find patients receiving oxygen-enhanced breathing mixtures while paper drapes, plastic endotracheal tubes, and electrical cautery are in use. Recently reviewed anesthetic and surgical malpractice cases have involved airway fires, combustion of surgical drapes, and facial fires from ignition near an oxygen mask or nasal cannula.

Although some operating room fires may be truly unpredictable and random occurrences, the allegation in resulting malpractice claims is bound to be that steps should have been taken to prevent them. From an anesthesiology standpoint, the most controllable variable is always the oxygen mixture delivered. Anesthesiologists named in claims involving fires may be called on to justify the indications for the use of oxygen at the time of the fire as well as their decisions regarding the flow of oxygen used.

Problems have arisen defending claims in which an anesthesiologist was using oxygen prophylactically on a sedation case while the patient's oxygen saturation was already high. An awareness of the risk of fire and communication between the surgeon and the anesthesiologist can ensure that oxygen is turned off when an ignition source is in use or that oxygen is switched to air to prevent stuffiness under the surgical drapes. Oxygen tends to pool under the drapes and may require time to disperse even when switched off.

When airway fires occur within the oropharynx, attention often focuses on whether an appropriate reinforced or laser endotracheal tube was used and whether there might have been an unnecessary oxygen leak. Reviewers of cases involving pediatric airway fires sometimes find that the oxygen delivered was actually in the adult range, many liters above the maximum minute ventilation of the child—possibly contributing to a large pooled oxygen leak. There will also likely be a determination of whether the endotracheal tube size was appropriate for the age of the child and whether the pressure at which the cuff leaked was quantified and documented by the anesthesiologist.

If a fire develops in the operating room, a quick response can help limit the injury to the patient. When possible, sterile water should be used to douse the fire. Oxygen should be immediately eliminated until the fire has been extinguished. Drapes and other flammables should be removed from the vicinity of the fire immediately. Airway fires will likely require the removal and replacement of the endotracheal tubes. Patients who have sustained airway fires should be carefully monitored postoperatively for respiratory difficulties *(5)*.

Newly Identified Risks

Although most of the risks of anesthesia have been known for decades, changes in perioperative techniques have added new risks, many of which have become apparent through the review of medical malpractice claims. Two of these risks, identified largely through reviews of adverse outcomes, are ischemic optic neuropathy in spine cases and respiratory arrests in sleep apnea patients after postoperative narcotics.

ISCHEMIC OPTIC NEUROPATHY

Ischemic optic neuropathy (ION) is the leading cause of blindness following general anesthesia. Depending on the surgical population, the incidence of ION has been estimated at between 0.1 and 1% (6). TDC has noted an increased incidence of claims involving postoperative blindness or severe visual impairment following spine surgeries in which controlled hypotension was utilized. Most of these cases involved an eventual diagnosis of ION (7).

ION is a visual impairment that results from inadequate oxygen delivery by the vessels supplying the optic nerve. It is classified as anterior or posterior, depending on which part of the nerve is affected. The two parts of the nerve have different blood supplies. Anterior ION typically spares central vision and causes peripheral visual field defects, whereas posterior ION, resulting from infarction in the central retinal artery, is usually associated with central visual defects (6). Because the anterior nerve is intraorbital, anterior ION can be caused by elevated intraorbital pressure, which could result from prolonged pressure against the eyes in patients who are facedown under general anesthesia. Posterior ION is seen most frequently in patients who have experienced hemodilution and hypotension, and it is the type more commonly found in spine cases using deliberate hypotension. Malpractice cases involving posterior ION have been successfully defended on the grounds that the anesthesiologist could not have improperly padded the patient's face because central retinal artery occlusion or anterior ION did not result.

In most postoperative cases reported, relative hypotension and anemia have contributed to the development of ION (6–10). It was felt by one author that although severe anemia alone might not cause ION, even a short episode of hypotension in an already anemic patient could predispose that patient to vision loss (10). The reasons for the recent increased incidence in ION are not entirely clear. New surgical techniques have made long spine surgeries more frequent, and cases in excess of 7 hours are not unusual. Long operating times do provide an opportunity for greater blood loss and longer periods of hypotension. There has also been a change in thinking regarding blood transfusion because of concerns about transmissible diseases. Although at one time a hemoglobin level of 10 g/dL was the commonly accepted threshold for intraoperative transfusion, many recommendations today suggest waiting for much lower hemoglobin levels or the development of unstable vital signs before transfusing. Because many of the affected patients were obese, it is possible that obesity itself is a factor—increasing abdominal compression while the patient is prone, elevating central venous pressure, and retarding venous drainage from the ophthalmic veins (7).

Risk management recommendations for the prevention of ION include the suggestion that anesthesiologists consider being more aggressive in transfusion practices for longer spine surgeries, possibly utilizing cell saver or predonated autologous blood (6,8,9). Anesthesiologists and surgeons should weigh the risks and benefits of the controlled hypotensive technique carefully and limit periods of extreme hypotension to crucial parts of the surgical procedure. Patients who have pre-existing hypertension, diabetes, atherosclerotic cardiovascular disease, or smoking histories are at higher risks for developing ION. Anesthesiologists should consider running mean arterial blood pressures higher in these patients. Accurate arterial line readings during the hypotensive period can help ensure that the blood pressure does not drop below an acceptable value. In prone cases, documenting on the anesthesia record at intervals that the face was frequently checked could go a long way toward proving that this was actually done. Patients suspected of developing ION should receive prompt ophthalmologic consultation (7).

SLEEP APNEA AND NARCOTIC POSTOPERATIVE PAIN MEDICATION

A number of malpractice cases reviewed by TDC involved postoperative respiratory arrests in patients with obstructive sleep apnea (OSA) who had received parenteral narcotics (11). Sleep apnea is a common disorder, with a prevalence of 1 to 4% in the middle-aged population (12,13). Affected patients are more likely to be obese, and there is a predominance of male OSA patients. Patients with sleep apnea have narrower upper airways that tend to collapse with normal rapid eye movement sleep. This tendency to obstruction is markedly increased by narcotic pain medication. OSA patients are much more sensitive to narcotic sedation than normal individuals (12,13). The effect of the narcotics on obstruction can be out of proportion to the level of sedation achieved (14). Many of these patients were described by nurses as complaining vociferously of pain before they fell asleep and obstructed to the point of cardiorespiratory arrest. Critical apneic episodes in these claims were observed with all routes of narcotic administration including intravenous and intramuscular injections, patient-controlled analgesia, and spinal and epidural administration.

Prevention of claims like these is complicated by the fact that not all patients with OSA carry the diagnosis preoperatively. Although OSA is diagnosable through formal sleep studies, it also has clinical hallmarks. These include loud snoring—often requiring couples to sleep in separate rooms; obstruction noted by the sleeping partner, including episodes of gasping and choking while asleep; and excessive daytime somnolence with an uncontrollable sleepiness interfering with professional or private life *(15)*. Patients who exhibit these symptoms might not all have OSA if evaluated by formal sleep studies, but it might be safer to treat them as if they did until proven otherwise *(11)*. Children with obstruction secondary to adenotonsillar hypertrophy may also have clinical sleep apnea presenting with the same clinical signs. They can also be at risk post-tonsillectomies if medicated with parenteral narcotics.

Risk-management suggestions include finding ways to monitor OSA patients appropriately postoperatively. Pulse oximetry currently has the ability to detect hypoxic episodes early, but oximeter alarms must be audible to hospital personnel if arrests are to be prevented. This can be accomplished in intensive care units or on wards that are staffed for this purpose. The administration of narcotics to OSA patients needs to be closely monitored. Pain medication orders for any given patient might be written by different individuals (e.g., surgeon, anesthesiologist, or primary care practitioner), not all of whom may be aware of the OSA diagnosis. Red-flagging the charts of OSA patients can warn all physicians and caregivers of the increased risk of narcotic administration.

Patients who use continuous positive airway pressure masks at home should be advised in advance to bring them to the hospital and should use them postoperatively where appropriate. As pain is treated more aggressively, the tragic complication of respiratory arrest in patients with OSA may be seen more frequently. Anesthesiologists should be alert to signs of OSA and should consider routinely asking questions to identify those patients at risk *(11)*.

When Bad Claims Happen to Good Anesthesiologists

Much has been written about the stress of being named in a malpractice lawsuit. Anesthesiologists may be particularly vulnerable in this circumstance because they do not have a consistent and loyal patient base and have only transient relationships with the other physicians with whom they work. As one anesthesiologist explained, "It's like you're only as good as your last case." Compounding the problem, the operating room is a small environment where bad news spreads rapidly, and the latest anesthetic misadventure may be fodder for locker room and lunchtime discussions for some time. The legal admonition not to speak to other physicians about the details of cases facing possible litigation can leave an anesthesiologist feeling isolated and alone.

However, in being sued, anesthesiologists are actually joining the ranks of the majority of their colleagues. One's partners are more likely than not to have been involved in malpractice cases themselves, but this is not a topic that comes up frequently for discussion in the operating room. Malpractice lawsuits are an unpleasant but real part of life for most anesthesiologists with busy practices. Those who manage to avoid litigation entirely are just as likely to be lucky as unusually skilled. With 4% of anesthesiology claims generated solely by surgical complications, avoiding those is really a matter of luck. Naturally, physicians tend to dwell on the facts of cases with adverse outcomes. In retrospect, it can be frustrating how simple the steps that would have avoided a complication might seem. However, any one anesthetic may be acceptably accomplished in many different ways, so there will always be a number of alternatives to whatever choices a physician makes. From a medical-legal standpoint, the standard of care does not depend on 20/20 hindsight but rather on what a similarly trained physician might have chosen to do given similar circumstances.

Ultimately, anesthesiologists are human. Errors in judgment or technique will be made, and sometimes patients will have ill effects that could possibly have been avoided. Anesthesia is certainly not risk-free, even in the best of hands, and complications will arise in every practice. As those who have lived through malpractice litigation attest, life goes on and operating room conversation ultimately shifts to more interesting topics. Rather than mulling over what they might have done wrong, anesthesiologists are encouraged to focus on the positive steps that can be taken to improve patient outcomes and enhance the defense of their own malpractice claims.

Preparing and keeping a detailed narrative of what occurred and becoming familiar with the medical record will enable an anesthesiologist to explain relevant issues to a defense attorney and malpractice company claims representative. Researching topics relevant to the case in anesthesiology texts and in literature available through Internet medical search engines like Medline® can help an attorney establish the standard of care and identify appropriate experts. It can also help to avoid being surprised by information discovered by the plaintiffs. From a risk-management standpoint, anesthesiologists should ask themselves honestly whether changing any of their routine practices could avoid similar complications in the future. Changing techniques after an untoward event in no way implies that what was done previously was substandard.

Many anesthesiologists describe feelings of depression or shame after serious complications occur or after receiving notification of an impending malpractice claim. Although initially it can seem like things will only get worse, the vast majority of physicians report that the negative feelings pass with time and life does return to normal. Spending time on outside activities they enjoy and avoiding overwork and sleep deprivation can only have positive effects on anesthesiologists' mental state and job function *(16)*.

REFERENCES

1. Lofsky AS. Guidelines for Risk Management in Anesthesiology, *TDC Anesthesia Handbook*, 1999.
2. Lofsky AS. Guidelines for Decreasing Dental Injury, *TDC Anesthesia Handbook*, 1999.
3. Lofsky AS: Labor and Delivery Disaster Claims, *TDC Risk Management Bulletin*, 2004.
4. Lofsky AS. Anesthesiology: A Claims Review Panel on Epidural Anesthesia, *TDC Anesthesia Handbook*, 1999.
5. Gorney M, Lofsky AS, Charles DM. Playing With Fire, *TDC Risk Management Advisory*, 2002.
6. Williams EL, Hart WM, Tempelhoff R. Postoperative Ischemic Optic Neuropathy. *Anesthesia and Analgesia* 1995;80:1018–1029.
7. Lofsky AS, Gorney M. Vision Problems after Spine Surgery With Controlled Hypotension. *TDC Risk Management Bulletin*, 1998.
8. Myers MA, Hamilton SR, Bogosian AJ, Smith CH, Wagner TA. Visual loss as a complication of spine surgery. Spine 1997;22(12):1325–1329.
9. Katz DM, Trobe ID, Cornblath WT, Kline LB. Ischemic optic neuropathy after lumbar spine surgery. Arch Opthalmol 1994;112:925–931.
10. Brown RH, Shauble JF, Miller NR. Anemia and hypotension as contributors to perioperative loss of vision. Anesthesiology 1994;80:222–226.
11. Lofsky AS. Sleep Apnea and Narcotic Postoperative Pain Medication: A Morbidity and Mortality Risk, *TDC Risk Management Bulletin*, 2001.
12. Tierney NM, Pollard BJ, Doran BR. Obstructive sleep apnoea. Anaesthesia 1989;44(3):235–237.
13. Boushra NN. Anaesthetic management of patients with sleep apnoea syndrome. Canadian J Anaesthesia 1996;43(6):599–616.
14. Esclamado RM, Glenn MG, McCulloch TM. Perioperative complications and risk factors in the surgical treatment of obstructive sleep apnea syndrome. Laryngoscope 1989;99(11):1125–1129.
15. Gentil B, Lienhart A, Fleury B. Enhancement of postoperative desaturation in heavy snorers. Anesthesia Analgesia 1995;81(2):389–392.
16. Lofsky AS. You Are Not Alone, *The Doctors' Advocate*, 2000.

11 Malpractice and Medical Practice

Obstetrics and Gynecology

Jack M. Schneider, MD

SUMMARY

This chapter presents general and specialty-specific issues leading to malpractice litigation. Strategies for decreasing medical error and preventing malpractice litigation are outlined with emphasis on accurate documentation, review of clinical information, selection and appropriate use of consultants, and above all, communication to the patient and family. The need to continue learning from national care guidelines and specialty-specific publications is emphasized.

Key Words: Labor; delivery; informed consent; maternal health care; Cesarean section; American College of Obstetrics and Gynecology Guidelines.

INTRODUCTION

Most cases of medical malpractice in obstetrics or gynecology follow from negligent performance of physician obligations that are not unique to this specialty. The physician must have the degree of learning and skill ordinarily possessed by reputable specialists practicing in the same field in the same or similar locality. Failure to meet these duties constitutes negligence, that is, the failure to meet the standard of care.

From: *Medical Malpractice: A Physician's Sourcebook*
Edited by: R. E. Anderson © Humana Press Inc., Totowa, NJ

These duties are not static and thereby require a commitment to continuing education. Meeting the standard of care requires knowledge and application of national professional (e.g., American College of Obstetricians and Gynecologists [ACOG]) guidelines (1) as well as pertinent knowledge set forth in specialty-related journal articles and other published works.

With the exception of the emergency situation, informed consent must be obtained from the patient or legal guardian prior to providing treatment or performing a procedure. Appropriate alternatives must be disclosed and the risks of the proposed intervention discussed in detail. Although possible death or serious bodily harm must be addressed, it is wise to discuss more common complications of the specific treatment and to present them in terms of expected frequency of occurrence. Guarantees should neither be stated nor implied.

The majority of suits regarding informed consent relate to two issues. One is failure to document the specific complications covered in the discussion (e.g., injury to the intestine requiring additional surgery). The other is failure to clearly define expectations. For example, the patient with pelvic pain often has the implied expectation of relief from the pain, but the physician knows this is possible but not certain.

Refusal by the patient to consent to a plan of treatment must be made on an informed basis. The physician should thoroughly document the advice provided, the patient's refusal to embrace the plan of care, and the potential consequences. It is extremely important that the practitioner not reflect his or her frustration or anger regarding the patient's expression of her right to refuse care. It is also important to have the patient sign in the medical record what specific aspect, or aspects, of the treatment is being refused.

When death or bodily harm results from a physician's failure to meet the standard of care, causation is established. If no harm inures from a standard-of-care issue, then there is typically no basis for suit. On the other hand, death or serious injury often leads to a malpractice suit even when negligence is not evident. The failure to communicate and to thoroughly document those conversations is the most frequent cause of litigation in obstetrics and gynecology. Communication is a two-way process, and the physician must be a good listener as well as presenter. I ascribe over 35 years of an active clinical practice of maternal and fetal medicine without litigation to open communication with my patients, their families, staff, and colleagues. In the cacophony of background noise, it is important to listen with clarity for the piccolo—in other words, what is really being said or not said by the patient and other interested parties. Importantly, communication includes body language. Ask the patient if she has any questions. Better still, ask her to explain her understanding of the point at issue.

Documentation of what you said to whom and their responses should be legible, accurate, concise, and without rancor. Additionally, it is the wise physician who timely reads the notes written by nurses and others with clarifying notations placed in the progress notes when there are differences of opinion.

When problems or complications occur and other specialists are involved, the original physician responsible for the woman's care must remain involved to provide continuity and coordination of care. The patient and her family expect that her doctor cares enough to see them and to explain what is happening.

Under the doctrine of standard of care, the responsible physician also has a duty to the patient to assure that consultants possess the degree of learning and skill possessed by reputable specialists providing consulting services in their area of expertise. The Ob/Gyn specialist should remain "captain of the ship" for his or her own patients. Consultants must be chosen with due care, and their care appropriately coordinated. The ACOG codified some of the medical conditions to consider for maternal and fetal medicine consultation (2). The responsible physician should define the expectations and scope of responsibility for the consultant. Consultants should provide timely follow-up and well-documented signoff of care.

Most consultants are not experts in the nuances of obstetrical- or gynecological-related complications or diseases. This makes it even more critical that the responsible Ob/Gyn specialist stay involved in his or her patient's care. Included in this responsibility is the review of radiology and laboratory data from the advantaged perspective of expertise in obstetrics and gynecology.

Spoliation of records is not only unethical but constitutes fraud, which is a criminal act. All alterations in the medical record should be lined through, dated, timed, and signed by the individual making the alteration.

Obstetric malpractice settlements are typically at the high end of payouts in that they involve care for both the mother and the child. Moreover, in the case of the damaged infant, many years of medical care and lost wages may need to be provided. The fact that obstetricians have two or more patients produces other unique medical liability considerations. Wrongful birth claims may entitle the parents to both economic and noneconomic damages. As an offset, the physician defendant can claim economic and noneconomic benefits such as love and happiness provided to the parents. Wrongful life litigation typically arises from negligent preconception care or from early pregnancy genetic counseling. The impaired child can claim economic but not noneconomic damages.

Care decisions involving the unborn child are often conflicted. On the one hand, the obstetrician has responsibility for both the mother and the fetus. However, the mother has the right and authority of ascribing patient status to her unborn under the doctrine of autonomy. Assuming a competent parent, the physician may only take those actions for the baby consented to by the mother/parent. All aspects of informed refusal should be thoroughly documented in the medical record, particularly the potential risks imparted to the unborn by the decision of the parent. It is best to avoid making the mother feel accused of potentially harming her baby.

The majority of malpractice claims in gynecology arise from the issues surrounding reproductive function. Both medical and surgical management of pelvic diseases may impair fertility and reproduction. When assisted reproduction is at issue, the learned Ob/Gyn specialist defers and refers to experts in the subspecialty of reproductive biology and endocrinology. For those physicians specializing in infertility, the majority of suits evolve from failure to meet implied outcome expectations. The patient has the right to receive informed consent, which includes outcome statistics comparing potential results from other infertility centers available to the patient.

The more common Ob/Gyn clinical issues leading to litigation include those inherent in all specialties, such as the following:

- Failure to provide informed consent.
- Failure to minimize the risk or extent of complications.
- Failure to provide emergent care in a timely manner.
- Failure to document the medical record.
- Failure to involve appropriate consultants in a timely manner.
- Failure to coordinate the patient's care and to keep the patient and family fully informed.

There are a number of issues specific to obstetrics and gynecology that are frequently the subject of litigation. Antibiotic prophylaxis is recommended to prevent vaginal cuff infection in all hysterectomies *(3)* and to prevent group B streptococcus (GBS) sepsis in the newborn *(4,5)*. The drug of choice for patients who have hysterectomies is a cephalosporin administered intravenously approx 30 minutes before transvaginal incision. For GBS prophylaxis, intravenous penicillin G is preferred over ampicillin for two reasons. A single loading dose of penicillin is likely as effective as two doses of ampicillin given 4 hours apart. In addition, the second most frequent cause of neonatal meningitis after GBS is *Escherichia coli*, which is often resistant to ampicillin.

Delayed diagnosis of cancer is another major issue for this specialty. The Ob/Gyn has a responsibility to inform, educate, and thus empower his or her patients about the importance of appropriate screening evaluations including mammography and Pap smears. The patient's history, including family history, is an important part of the assessment of risk. Trust the patient when she notes a change in status and listen to the history she relates. The responsible physician best serves the patient when he or she obtains the history in the patient's "own words" rather than the secondhand interpretation of staff's documentation. A family history of breast cancer, particularly under age 45 years, imparts increased risk to the patient. Physical examination should include the axillary lymph nodes. Suspicious mammograms may be clarified with a diagnostic sonogram. All suspicious masses should be biopsied, regardless of the mammogram interpretation.

The diagnosis of cervical cancer is an important consideration in the evaluation of intravaginal bleeding. Pelvic sonography in the postmenopausal patient may be done to assess the thickness of the endometrium. Again, the patient's history is often telling and may lead to a diagnosis of cancer when the appropriate evaluations are performed.

The other major area of liability for this specialty is prenatal care and delivery. Prenatal diagnostic ultrasonographic evaluation of the fetus is an increasing area of litigation. It is essential that the responsible Ob/Gyn clarify for the patient what fetal anatomy can or cannot be seen and what diagnoses can or cannot be made. Limitations of equipment, the impact of fetal position and number, and maternal size should be emphasized. For example, only one-third of major fetal anatomic abnormalities are defined at second-trimester scans. Even when a consultant provides the interpretation of the study, the primary Ob/Gyn should review the implications of the findings with the patient and family. Additionally, genetic counseling is now so complex that only a certified counselor should do it.

Fetal death imparts a responsibility on the part of the delivering physician for documentation of the gross anatomy of the baby, the umbilical cord, and the placenta. Such descriptors are far more meaningful than those following examination by the pathologist hours to days later.

Autopsy of the dead fetus should be encouraged even when it appears grossly normal. The bulk of suits for wrongful fetal death arise when the death is unexplained, although up to 75% of fetal deaths can be understood after thorough gross, microscopic, and genetic analyses *(6)*. The obstetric department should define a protocol to assess all fetal deaths.

Much potential litigation can be prevented by the responsible Ob/Gyn discussing all findings with the patient and her family. This review should take place prior to discharge from the hospital and again at the postpartum visit. Under no circumstances should the patient be left with unanswered questions or concerns as these only drive attempts to get explanations from an attorney.

Complications of induction of labor, although not very common, do occur and have associated risks to mother and, more commonly, baby. Informed consent should be obtained according to ACOG Practice Bulletin regarding induction of labor *(7)*. Elements of the consent include the indication for the induction, the agents and methods of labor stimulation, the risks attendant to the use of these agents, methods and alternatives (typically expectant management or Cesarean section [C-section]), and the associated risk for mother and baby. It is noteworthy that the bulletin states, "A physician capable of performing a Cesarean delivery should be readily available." Fetal gestational age should be defined and confirmed by sonography early in the pregnancy to preclude induction of labor for a premature infant. It is recommended that all patients undergoing labor induction have electronic fetal heart rhythm and uterine contraction monitoring although its utility is problematic except in the high-risk pregnancy.

Electronic fetal heart rate (FHR) monitoring is a classic example of a procedure becoming codified as the standard of care without proof of effectiveness. In fact, the prevalence of cerebral palsy has not been altered by this modality *(8)*. The physician must be certain that he or she and the nurses are using the same terminology in describing the FHR tracing. For example, quantification of variability is subjective, and there is no such terminology as late variables—indeed variable decelerations are so named in part because the timing of the deceleration to the uterine contraction varies in its onset, including occurring late. Just as important, the physician should review the nurses' notes with special attention to the terminology used, contact times, information given to the physician, and the physician's responses.

Particular emphasis should be placed on the review of the initial, admission FHR tracing to ascertain whether or not the tracing should be characterized as reassuring. The previously damaged fetus, now with recovered acid–base status, may demonstrate a reassuring tracing. A nonreassuring tracing, particularly with little or no baseline variability, does highly correlate with a neurologically injured fetus. Other assessors of fetal well-being (e.g., the biophysical profile, scalp pH, arterial O_2 saturation, and APGAR scores) are no more predictive than the FHR tracing of the neurologic status of the fetus and newborn. The umbilical cord gases correlate well with neurological injury in the newborn, but they must be assessed immediately after birth. Following neonatal resuscitation, respiratory gas values typically show a more severe metabolic acidosis than is evident at the time of birth. Accordingly, umbilical cord gases should be obtained in all depressed or resuscitation-requiring newborns.

Hypoxic-ischemic encephalopathy (HIE) injury pattern in the newborn must be placed in perspective with all the known pertinent clinical information. As noted, the FHR tracing should be reviewed in its entirety. After dealing with the emergent situation, all actions taken or not taken should be clearly documented in the medical record along with explanations provided to the parents. Communication with the baby's physician is very important not only to clarify the timing of the baby's neurological injury but also to facilitate the obstetrician's translation of the baby's status to the mother and family.

Shoulder dystocia is not predictable and generally not preventable. The associations with maternal factors are weak except for an expulsive resolution to the second stage of labor and fetal macrosomia often seen in cases of maternal diabetes. Even making the diagnosis of macrosomia is difficult, and late pregnancy sonography is no better than clinical guesstimate. Elective induction of labor or elective C-section delivery for women suspected of carrying a macrosomic fetus is generally not recommended. On the other hand, the case has been made for elective C-section when the estimated fetal weight exceeds 4500 g in women with diabetes.

It is essential to review the nurses' notes to ascertain their concordance with your own notes on clinical events. For example, it is not uncommon for the nurse's notes to reflect the use of fundal pressure rather than suprapubic pressure. Although there are no data to support the use of one maneuver over another, the McRobert's patient positioning is simple and resolves about 50% of the cases of anterior shoulder impaction. Fundal pressure prior to the diagnosis of shoulder dystocia is not a standard-of-care issue. Cervical plexus injury has been reported without documented shoulder dystocia at the time of vaginal birth *(9)* as well as at the time of planned C-section *(10).*

Fracture of the clavicle occurs frequently with vaginal birth and does not reflect negligence. There is no scientific basis that all or even most brachial plexus injuries result from inappropriate maneuvers at delivery (11).

Newborn seizure activity is so rare following delivery with shoulder dystocia that intracerebral hemorrhage must be ruled out. HIE with mental retardation and/or cerebral palsy is also rare (<1%), unless the time from diagnosis of dystocia at delivery of the head to resuscitation exceeds 10 minutes. Video recording during periods of obstetric emergencies should not be allowed. Although the severity of the dystocia cannot be defined as mild, moderate, or severe, a videotape is often very revealing as to the twists and turns exerted on the baby's neck. Documentation of the sequence and timing of the maneuvers is critical as are APGAR scores, need for resuscitation, and evident plexus injury.

Obstetric hemorrhage is the most common cause of maternal death when associated complications are included. Death secondary to hemorrhage would be most unusual in a modern obstetric service in the United States. Accepted risk factors include delays in identification of the site of the bleeding and in volume resuscitation with appropriate blood products. This often follows a failure to appreciate the quantity of blood the obstetric patient can lose before exhibiting shock followed rapidly by cardiovascular collapse and the morbidity of associated organ injury. Furthermore, tachycardia ($\geq$110 bpm) and systolic hypotension ($\leq$90 mmHg) tend to be late signs in the obstetric patient occurring typically after a volume loss of approx 40%. Orthostatic systolic blood pressure checking is a more reliable indicator of significant hypovolemia—a 10 mmHg decrease equating in pregnancy to a deficit of 1 L or more.

The medical management of obstetric hemorrhage, particularly with uterine atony, includes oxytocic agents such as oxytocin, methylergonovine, Hemabate™ intrauterine, and misoprostal per rectum. Blood products are preferred over crystalloid (12). Fibrinogen replacement is almost always required because the more common antecedents to the hemorrhage are defibrination associated with placental abruption, dead fetus syndrome, or amniotic fluid embolism.

Surgical interventions are often not useful. Ligation of the internal hypogastric arteries does not improve survival (13). On the other hand, ligation of the ovarian and uterine pedicles without vessel transection may significantly decrease blood loss (12). Hysterectomy in the face of uncontrollable bleeding typically adds to the blood loss as well as the intraoperative and postoperative complications. Packing, oversewing the placental bed, and suture techniques such as the B-Lynch suture *(12,14)* may slow blood loss sufficiently to allow adequate fluid resuscitation before proceeding with hysterectomy or other surgical interventions. Use of antishock trousers (MAST) may prove a lifesaving procedure.

Massive hemorrhage (i.e., poststabilization hematocrit ≤15%) in the obstetric patient poses significant risk for subsequent pulmonary embolism. For this reason, heparin therapy should be considered after the patient is without evident bleeding *(12)*.

The postdates pregnancy, defined as at least 42 weeks of gestation, is associated with an increased risk of central nervous system (CNS) injury in the fetus. Early pregnancy definition of gestational dating is paramount to avoid overdiagnosis of postdate pregnancy or the failure to effect delivery when the diagnosis is evident. Most practitioners obtain serial nonstress tests (NST) and amniotic fluid volume assessments to evaluate fetal well-being. The latter is more predictive of neurological injury than the NST. A diagnosis of oligohydramnios should prompt delivery by induction of labor to the extent that the fetus is tolerant of the uterine contractions. Again, reviewing the FHR tracing from the time of admission is important to assess fetal well-being. Most instances of meconium aspiration and CNS injury in these pregnancies occur *in utero* and usually do not reflect negligence.

The delivering physician should describe both the quantity and quality (meconium: thickness and color) of the amniotic fluid as well as the umbilical cord, the membranes, placenta, and baby regarding meconium staining, loss of subcutaneous fat, and dry, sloughing skin.

Operative delivery by the vaginal route must meet defined criteria, and these should be documented in the medical record *(15)*. Multiple attempts at operative delivery, plus use of both forceps and the vacuum extractor significantly increase the risk for CNS injury to the infant *(16)*.

Delivery by planned C-section requires informed consent to include a defensible indication for the procedure. In the case of the emergency situation, the obstetrician should carry out only essential steps to effect delivery. Intrabladder catheter placement, presurgery sponge count, suction apparatus, and cautery setup all waste valuable time. There should be a slimmed down operative tray with no sponges. All emergency intra-abdominal procedures mandate a postoperative abdominal film to rule out a retained sponge.

There are many variables that impact the neurologic outcome for the baby, which explains why some babies born after a 30-minute time delay do well, whereas others born after 15 minutes do not. The 30-minute rule of decision for C-section and incision for delivery does not ensure protection for the baby. Again, communication with the baby's physician is essential to define to the extent possible the cause and timing of the newborn injury.

Vaginal birth after prior C-section requires informed consent and the meeting of defined standards (17). Notably, ACOG states that a physician must be immediately available throughout active labor and be capable of monitoring labor and performing an emergency Cesarean delivery. The risk of uterine rupture does not preclude the induction of labor, but the induction requires careful, continuous monitoring. When the obstetrician documents any emergency responses, he or she should note any time difference on the clock in the labor suite and the operating room. Ideally, all clocks used for time keeping should be synchronized.

All patients with hypertension complicating pregnancy should be evaluated by an obstetrician at the hospital for evidence of complications. Emergency department staff, including physicians, is generally not sufficiently sensitive to the subtleties of diseases complicating pregnancy.

Thromboembolic disease is a common complication of pregnancy, particularly following pelvic surgery. A family history of early age of onset or recurrent thromboembolism suggests an inherited thrombophilia. This may be associated with increased risk for thromboses in the fetus and newborn (12).

Turning to surgical areas of liability, losing a laparotomy sponge in the abdomen is rarely defensible. Placing a sponge in the gutters to absorb blood reflects a lack of understanding that adhesions follow injury to the peritoneum (as may occur from abrasions caused by the sponge), not the blood. If blood in the pelvis caused adhesions, the ovulating female would have adherence of her ovaries to contiguous tissues. A ring or other instrument should be used to mark all sponges. An abdominal film should be obtained following emergency abdominal surgery and in all instances of a reported incorrect sponge count.

Recently, many gynecological issues leading to litigation have reflected advances in technology. Foremost among these is the use of the laparoscope for diagnostic and/or therapeutic surgical procedures. Informed consent should address the patient's expectations. For example, pelvic pain is seldom significantly lessened with the lysis of adhesions unless the adhesions are associated with a subacute inflammatory process. Indeed, adhesions are best left alone unless lysis is required to access diseased organs, because after surgery, the lysed adhesions simply reform. An increase in the number of lysis procedures increases the risk of organ injury including bowel and also increases the risk of subsequent bowel obstruction. Lysing adhesions to "just do something" is often unwise. If not specifically covered by the informed consent, then adhesions should be left alone.

The prudent practitioner will not hesitate to convert to an open procedure when adhesions limit exposure. Injury to the bowel may be secondary to a needle puncture or sharp or thermal dissection. When recognized at the time of surgery, the gynecologist should be able to effect a satisfactory repair.

The patient with bowel injury not recognized at the time of surgery typically presents to the emergency department 36–48 hours following discharge with complaints of fever, nausea, vomiting, and abdominal pain. The gynecologist must not rely on the emergency department or office staff to determine the patient's status and most likely diagnosis. The patient should be evaluated by the responsible gynecologist to ensure that early, aggressive management of sepsis is undertaken, thus forestalling septic shock with its high rates of morbidity and mortality.

Patient selection for hysterectomy should be very carefully done with focus on the patient's health and age. There are many alternatives to hysterectomy, which must be covered in the informed consent process. It may be negligent to do a hysterectomy in a high-risk patient when an endometrial ablation procedure would have sufficed. Again, prophylactic antibiotics for hysterectomy are the standard of care.

Injury of contiguous organs may occur and not be reflective of negligent care. However, failure to recognize the importance of certain postoperative signs and/or symptoms may constitute negligence. Bladder and bowel injury should be recognized at the time of the gynecologic procedure and appropriate repair should be undertaken. Wound infection and dehiscence risk is minimized by avoiding the use of a nonisotonic cleansing solution and by the use of a transverse incision. Drains should not be sewn in place to avoid a nidus for abscess formation.

Anesthesia approaches are significantly influenced by the physiology of pregnancy and fetal pharmacokinetics. In general, inhalation agents used with general anesthesia do not pose risk for the fetus as long as the ambient O_2 is maintained at normal levels. Failed intubation is more common in pregnant patients particularly in late pregnancy, with short stature and with the generalized edema of preeclampsia (18).

The maternal mortality rate with general anesthesia for C-section is significantly higher than with epidural, but this likely reflects, at least in part, the emergency at hand that prompted use of inhalation anesthesia *(19)*.

Regional anesthesia is the preferred labor and delivery analgesia approach unless contraindicated because of maternal conditions. It is important to maintain adequate maternal cardiac output and thus uteroplacental perfusion to optimize gas exchange by the fetus.

REFERENCES

1. American College of Obstetricians and Gynecologists. Compendium of selected publications. Washington, DC; ACOG, 2003.
2. American Academy of Pediatrics, American College of Obstetricians and Gynecologists. 5th Ed. Elk Grove Village, IL: AAP; Washington, DC: ACOG, 2002: 365–368.
3. American College of Obstetricians and Gynecologists. Antibiotic prophylaxis for gynecologic procedures. ACOG Practice Bulletin 23. Washington, DC:ACOG, 2001.
4. American College of Obstetricians and Gynecologists. Prevention of early-onset group B streptococcal disease in newborns. ACOG Committee Opinion 279. Washington, DC: ACOG, 2002.
5. Prevention of Perinatal Group B Streptococcal Disease—Revised Guidelines from CDC. MMWR 2002;151(R11):1–22.
6. Fretts RC, Boyd ME, Usher HA. The changing pattern of fetal death, 1961–1988. Obstet Gynecol 1992;79:35–39.
7. American College of Obstetricians and Gynecologists. Induction of labor. ACOG Practice Bulletin 10. Washington, DC: ACOG, 1999.
8. Clark SI, Hankins GDV. Temporal and demographic trends in cerebral palsy—fact or fiction. AM J Obstet Gynecol 2003;188:628–633.
9. Gherman RB, Ouzounian JG, Miller DA, Kwok L, Goodwin TM. Spontaneous vaginal delivery: a risk factor for Erb's palsy? Am J Obstet Gynecol 1998;178: 423–427.
10. Gherman RB, Goodwin TM, Ouzounian JG, Miller DA, Paul RH. Brachial plexus palsy associated with cesarean section: An *in utero* injury? Am J Obstet Gynecol 1997;177:1162–1164.
11. Sandmire HF, DeMott, RK. Erb's palsy: concepts of causation. Obstet Gynecol 2000;95:941,942.
12. Schneider JM. Hemorrhage: Related Obstetric and Medical Disorders. In: Bonica JJ, McDonald J S, eds. Principles and Practice of Obstetric Analgesia and Anesthesia, 2nd Ed. Malvern, PA: Williams & Wilkins, 1995:865–917.
13. Evans S, McShane P. The efficacy of internal iliac artery ligation in obstetric hemorrhage. Surg Gynecol Obstet 1985;160:250–253.
14. Smith KL, Basket TF. Uterine compression sutures as an alternative to hysterectomy for severe postpartum hemorrhage. J Obstet Gynaecol Can 2003;25(3):197–200.
15. American College of Obstetricians and Gynecologists. Operative vaginal delivery. ACOG Practice Bulletin 17. Washington, DC: ACOG, 2000.

16. Towner D, Castro MA, Eby-Wilkens E, Gilbert WM. Effect of mode of delivery in nulliparous women on neonatal intracranial injury. N Engl J Med 1999;341: 1709–1714.
17. American College of Obstetricians and Gynecologists. Vaginal birth after previous cesarean delivery. ACOG Practice Bulletin 5. Washington, DC:ACOG, 1999.
18. Barnardo PD, Jenkins JG. Failed tracheal intubation in obstetrics: a 6-year review in the UK region. Anesthesia 2000;55:690–694.
19. Hawkins JL, Koonin LM, Palmer SK, Gibbs CP. Anesthesia-related deaths during obstetric delivery in the United States 1979–1990. Anesthesiology 1997; 86:277–284.

12 Breast Cancer Litigation

Richard E. Anderson, MD, FACP
and David B. Troxel, MD, FACP

SUMMARY

Breast cancer is the most common diagnosis in medical malpractice claims in the United States. This chapter analyzes 100 consecutive breast cancer claims from The Doctors Company, a large national medical malpractice insurer. Factors that contribute to this high claims frequency include patient discovery of the breast mass, delay in diagnosis, mammography communication errors, patient age, tumor size, and tumor stage. The potential for computer-aided detection to reduce mammography interpretation errors is discussed. Finally, pathology claims involving breast biopsy and fine needle aspiration are analyzed and strategies are presented to minimize diagnostic error.

Key Words: Breast cancer; breast cancer malpractice; breast cancer claims; mammography error; breast biopsy error; breast fine needle aspiration.

BREAST CANCER LITIGATION:
THE CLINICAL CONTEXT

Breast cancer is the most common diagnosis in malpractice claims in the United States. There are many reasons for this *(1)*.

From: *Medical Malpractice: A Physician's Sourcebook*
Edited by: R. E. Anderson © Humana Press Inc., Totowa, NJ

- Breast cancer is a common disease.
- The public has been educated to believe that early detection of cancer guarantees a good outcome.
- Breast cancer is an emotionally charged diagnosis that not only threatens life but also acutely challenges self-image and affects women of all ages.
- Seventy-five percent of women with breast cancer have no known risk factors, so the diagnosis is nearly always a shock.
- It is commonly the patient who first discovers a mass, so she is acutely aware when prompt diagnosis is not undertaken.
- The preponderance of evidence suggests screening mammography reduces breast cancer mortality by 25–30% in women age 50 years and older. The magnitude of benefit is less clear in younger women, yet the majority of malpractice claims involve women younger than age 50.

This chapter reviews the clinical circumstances surrounding breast cancer litigation. We then analyze in detail the liability faced by pathologists in dealing with breast biopsies.

Although there is some comfort in the fact that few cases involve physician incompetence or technical inadequacy, this is no solace to the patient and does not form the basis of a strong defense in court. The vast majority of cases allege delay in diagnosis, and these claims may be divided into those involving diagnostic error and those involving poor communication. Additional claims arise from therapeutic acts of omission or commission.

Breast cancer is a common disease, and most women are familiar with the cumulative incidence figure that one in nine American women will have breast cancer in her lifetime. Although this figure is accurate, it is somewhat misleading because it includes precursor *in situ* lesions that have not yet become cancers and assumes that women will live to age 80 years or older and not die from other causes before that age. The prevalence of the disease is increasing because of the wide use of mammographic screening and the aging of the population (the incidence rises with age). Most breast cancers present without symptoms, and it is the patient herself who most often discovers the tumor; therefore, any delay in diagnosis is both readily apparent and unlikely to be excused.

The Doctors Company (TDC), a national physician-owned medical malpractice insurance company, analyzed 100 closed claims involving breast cancer in an attempt to identify repetitive problems *(2–4)*. This is, to our knowledge, the largest single-source breast cancer claims study ever undertaken. Closed claims were reviewed to ensure the full range of outcome data would be available. Consecutive files were chosen to evaluate all actual case presentations independent of outcome.

Overall Outcomes

The 100 consecutive files involved 80 individual patients with breast cancer. In these cases, 127 physicians were defendants and 42 (33%) ultimately paid indemnity. Of the 80 women, 36 (45%) were successful against at least one defendant physician. Four claims went to trial and two resulted in a verdict for the plaintiff.

Presenting Symptoms

Clinical findings on presentation were documented in 71 cases. Of these, there were 34 cases with no symptoms. A palpable lump was found in 28 cases, pain was present in 8 cases, and there was nipple discharge in 1 case.

Discovery of the Mass

Frequently, the patient discovers her own breast cancer. In this series, the patient made the initial finding of a mass in 33 of 46 (72%) cases where the initial discovery was clearly documented. The average indemnity in this group was $350,000. In the 13 cases where the physician initially detected the mass, the average indemnity was $156,538.

Overall, TDC closes more than 80% of its claims without any indemnity payment (5). When cases go to trial, TDC gains a defense verdict four of of five times. However, with breast cancer claims, the defense prevails less often. In this study, indemnity was paid on behalf of the defendant physician 33% of the time, and overall, 45% of breast cancer plaintiffs received payment from at least one physician defendant. The fact that the patient herself so frequently discovers the mass is an important part of the reason for this difference, because any delay in the ultimate diagnosis of cancer is apparent. Moreover, it is the patient herself who has brought the problem to the physician's attention, so it is difficult to excuse unnecessary delay. Therefore, it is not surprising that indemnity payments are considerably higher where the patient rather than the doctor initially detects the tumor ($350,000 vs $156,538). When the physician discovers the tumor, it is more likely that the patient has contributed to any delay in diagnosis.

Physician Specialties

Doctors in nearly all specialties see patients with breast cancer, but the litigation burden falls most heavily on those charged with making

Exposure Count by Specialty

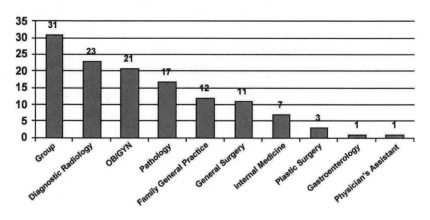

Fig. 1. Breast cancer litigation by specialty *(5)*.

the initial diagnosis. Radiologists who read the mammograms, pathologists who read the biopsies, and obstetricians/gynecologists who frequently provide primary care for women are the specialists most frequently sued (*see* Fig. 1).

Mammography

It appears that many patients believe that screening mammography should either prevent the disease or guarantee a cure if it is found. The likelihood that an individual screening mammogram will reveal malignancy is between 1 in 200 and 1 in 250 *(5a)*. This makes finding the one true positive study difficult, but gives patients an exaggerated sense of the protective effect of screening.

Mammograms are involved in the majority of breast cancer cases and are the most common source of malpractice claims against radiologists. Allegations can be divided into two broad areas: communication and interpretation. Communication errors involve transmittal of correctly interpreted findings and are usually obvious and problematic. Interpretation issues are more complex.

Mammography was performed in 77 of the 80 patients in the TDC study, and in 30 patients, the mammogram was pivotal to the outcome of the claim. What was unexpected is that interpretation error was the key factor in only 9 claims (30%). The high frequency of allegations of misinterpretation by the radiologist can be explained by several factors.

- The inherent difficulty in interpreting the complex and often non-specific findings, particularly in women under age 40 (reading a mammogram has been likened to detecting a snowball in a blizzard).
- Wide ranges in detection sensitivity even among experienced radiologists.
- The absence of an alternative nonsurgical gold standard for definitive diagnosis.
- The difficulty of balancing the serious consequences of a false-negative reading with the consequences of a false-positive reading that leads to a negative biopsy (attendant anxiety, surgical morbidity, and cost).

Currently, mammograms have a cancer-detection sensitivity of approx 80%. This means that one in five cancers will not be detected on a mammogram, either because it is simply not visible (radiographic false-negative) or because the radiologist fails to see it or sees it but incorrectly interprets it as benign (physician error).

Large studies show that radiologists vary by as much as 40% in their ability to detect mammographically visible cancers. In one study, prior mammograms were reviewed retrospectively and 54% indicated the presence of a lesion that might have been interpreted as suspicious for cancer (6). Of these, however, 44% would still have been labeled negative if read in a blinded fashion.

The remaining 70% of the mammogram-related claims in the TDC study involved communication error, and nearly all were preventable. In these cases, there was a failure to carry a correct radiographic interpretation of possible cancer through the necessary steps that lead to a definitive diagnosis. Despite the myriad pressures of daily medical practice, such lapses are difficult to defend in court. The clinical circumstances of these lapses vary from case to case, and in some the patient bore significant responsibility; however, in each instance a positive mammography finding did not receive appropriate attention. Given the fact that even in the best of hands and using the best available equipment, 15–20% of breast cancers will not be detected by screening mammography, it is critical to institute measures to eliminate these preventable errors.

Delay in Diagnosis

The majority of claims involving breast cancer involve allegations of delayed diagnosis. However, to be successful a malpractice claim must prove more than a breach in the standard of care that resulted in later diagnosis. It must also be shown that the patient suffered harm as a result of the delay. If the delay is long enough for the cancer to metastasize, the harm is apparent because metastatic breast cancer is essentially incurable.

In this series, only 1 of the 80 claimants had metastatic disease at the time of initial diagnosis. In the other 79 cases, inferences about potential harm were made from the size of the cancer and the status of the regional lymph nodes at the time of actual diagnosis compared to their hypothetical status at the time of "missed" diagnosis. The critical variable in all delayed diagnosis cases is time. How long was the alleged delay?

Ten litigated cases alleged delays of less than 6 months; 9 of 10 of these cases were won by the defense. This seems a surprisingly large number of claims alleging such a short period of delay. There are several potential explanations:

- If the patient is the initial discoverer of the lump, she may resent even very brief "delays" in definitive diagnosis.
- There is widespread confusion among nonphysicians about the difference between early diagnosis and prevention. Too often, patients undergoing annual mammography believe that they should not get breast cancer at all.
- Breast cancer is a serious misfortune for anyone. In our society, there is an increasingly widespread belief that all adversity should be compensated.

Most often, the alleged delay was between 6 and 24 months; these were defended successfully in 25 of 39 claims (64%). This is a clinical "gray area," where it is usually difficult to determine with certainty the actual effect of delay on prognosis. Competent witnesses for the plaintiff and defense are likely to disagree on the impact of the delay on outcome.

Beyond 24 months, longer delays do not necessarily mean higher awards although the causation argument (e.g., that the alleged delay did not matter) is harder to make. Delays beyond 24 months resulted in plaintiff awards 6 of 13 times (46%). Only a few cases involved delays of longer than 5 years, and these are often the result of patients lost to follow-up in circumstances in which they bear much of the responsibility.

Tumor Size

Tumors larger than 2 cm at diagnosis were preponderant (27 cases), and tumors 5 cm or greater were the single most frequent category (17 cases). Indemnity in paid claims seems to increase with larger tumors. Only a single claim involved a cancer smaller than 1 cm. The size of the

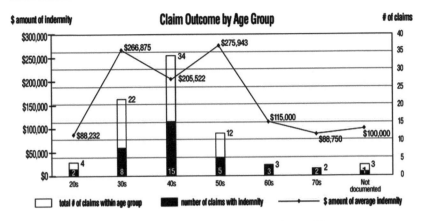

Fig. 2. Breast cancer litigation and age (5).

tumors in these claims is larger than that seen in a population that receives regular mammographic screening. There are several hypotheses to explain this observation:

- Clinically advanced cases are more likely to be litigated.
- Mammographic screening is underutilized.
- Tumors with rapid growth rates are likely to be larger at initial diagnosis.

Lymph Node Status

The majority of claims involved patients with positive axillary lymph nodes; within this group, the majority had four or more involved nodes. Cases involving positive nodes resulted in indemnity payment in 25 of 43 cases (58%). This is a higher than expected percentage of high-stage presentations at initial diagnosis and suggests that the litigation process is selecting relatively advanced cases for adjudication. There are a number of potential explanations for this finding.

- Patients with higher stage disease can more readily prove damages and thus are more likely to litigate.
- It is possible that litigation selects for a subset of aggressive, fast-growing cancers.
- In some cases, the patient was lost to follow-up through no fault of the physician.
- It is likely, that a significant percentage of these patients did receive suboptimal care.

Patient Age

The age of the patient is important (*see* Fig. 2.). The majority of breast cancer claims, and the highest indemnities, involves premenopausal women. Indemnity was paid in 25 of 60 (42%) cases involving women under age 50. Four claims involved women in their 20s, an age when breast cancer may not be the first diagnosis that comes to mind and when screening mammography is infrequently performed. The younger the patient, the easier it is to demonstrate significant damages from lost wages, the costs of raising young children, and lost child-bearing potential. Although the index of suspicion for breast cancer in very young women may be lower, the impact of missing the diagnosis is especially high. Because the insensitivity of mammography in women younger than age 40 is well-recognized, clinical follow-up is mandatory and making a definitive diagnosis is essential. There were fewer claims for older women, but 10 of 17 (59%) paid indemnity.

BREAST BIOPSY AND THE MICROSCOPIC DIAGNOSIS OF BREAST CANCER

We turn now to an analysis of the clinical and medical-legal issues surrounding the microscopic diagnosis of breast cancer.

In a separate study of pathology claims, TDC reviewed 218 consecutive surgical pathology and fine needle aspiration (FNA) claims from 1995 to 1997 *(7–9)*. Breast FNA accounted for 6% of these claims and breast biopsy accounted for another 14%. When claims involving breast FNA, breast biopsy, and breast frozen section were combined, breast specimens accounted for 22% of all pathology claims. Fifty-four percent of breast biopsy claims involved the false-negative diagnosis of breast carcinoma, whereas 35% were for the false-positive diagnosis of carcinoma.

Breast Fine Needle Aspiration

A false-negative breast FNA usually results from the failure to adequately sample a breast mass (sampling error) and is responsible for the majority of claims. Often, these claims involve a woman with a palpable breast mass, in whom an FNA is negative, and who is subsequently diagnosed with carcinoma. In many of these cases, an FNA diagnosis of "fibrocystic change" or "negative" was made on sparsely cellular smears. Although the definition of breast FNA specimen adequacy is controversial *(10–12)*, it is important to remember that many physicians perform FNA procedures infrequently and lack formal training in smear preparation technique. For this reason, they are often unable to reliably assess whether or not the mass was adequately sampled. Therefore, when the slides have only a few cells, it is hazardous for a pathologist to assume that the specimen is a representative sample and proceed to make a diagnosis of fibrocystic change or negative. This is a special problem in a managed care environment where patients frequently change health plans—and physicians—and are often lost to follow-up. Most of these claims could have been prevented if the diagnosis had been "nondiagnostic because of sparse cellularity, additional diagnostic studies recommended." Under these circumstances, most clinicians would repeat the FNA or proceed to excisional or needle biopsy and the correct diagnosis would be made promptly.

Triple Test Strategy

Every breast FNA report should include a statement reminding the clinician that breast FNA has a false-negative rate of 3–5% and a false-positive rate of 0.5–2%. The consequences of these errors can be minimized by applying the triple test strategy, that is, correlating the FNA results with the mammogram/ultrasound findings and the clinical breast examination and performing a biopsy if these are discordant. Whenever possible, the pathologist should review the mammogram and ultrasound reports and discuss the physical findings with the clinician before releasing the FNA report. If the pathologist knows there is triple test discordance, then this should be stated in the report and biopsy recommended. This strategy would eliminate most liability claims for breast FNA and result in improved clinical outcomes.

Claims resulting from false-positive FNAs usually are caused by interpretation errors. Most commonly, an FNA diagnosis of carcinoma is made on a mass subsequently shown to be a fibroadenoma. The claim results from either unnecessary mastectomy or axillary node sampling if breast conservation is elected. In almost every instance, these claims would have been prevented if the triple test strategy had been applied.

Breast Biopsy

Some breast biopsy claims involve the differentiation of low-grade ductal carcinoma *in situ* (DCIS) from ductal involvement by lobular carcinoma *in situ* (LCIS). This differentiation can be difficult and is often subjective. It is hoped that the use of immunostains for E-cadherin will add objectivity to this distinction *(13,14)*. Occasional claims involve the differentiation of DCIS from atypical duct hyperplasia (ADH). This is not surprising, because poor interobserver reproducibility in the diagnosis of ductal proliferative lesions is well documented even among experts *(15–17)*.

In each of these scenarios, misdiagnosis can result in patient injury. DCIS is a premalignant lesion that may be treated surgically to obtain negative margins and sometimes with radiation therapy or mastectomy. In contrast, LCIS and ADH are regarded as "markers" for increased risk involving both breasts and are usually managed conservatively by surveillance alone. When considering a diagnosis of DCIS, LCIS, or ADH, it is important to keep these management differences in mind.

Many primary care clinicians (and some surgeons) do not fully understand the terms DCIS, LCIS, ADH, and atypical lobular hyperplasia (ALH). For this reason, the pathology report should include an explanation of the clinical significance of these terms, that is, that DCIS is a premalignant lesion placing the biopsied breast at risk, whereas LCIS and atypical hyperplasia are "markers" for risk in both breasts. It is also important to state clearly that there is no invasive carcinoma, because the "carcinoma" in DCIS or LCIS may be misunderstood to mean the patient has "cancer." These are confusing terms and should be explained in the pathology report to avoid miscommunication and prevent inappropriate management decisions.

Nineteen percent of all breast biopsy claims involved large-core (cutting) needle biopsies of palpable breast masses or stereotaxic image-guided needle biopsies of nonpalpable lesions discovered on mammography. The following is a list of some diagnostic errors uncovered in a review of these claims:

1. The misdiagnosis of DCIS, sclerosing adenosis, and florid adenosis as invasive ductal carcinoma. Injury results if mastectomy is performed without first performing an excisional biopsy of the lesion or if axillary lymph nodes are sampled at the time an excisional biopsy is performed.
2. The misdiagnosis of LCIS involving ducts as low-grade DCIS. Because LCIS is a "marker" for increased risk, whereas DCIS is a premalignant lesion, the management is totally different. Patient injury results if axillary lymph node sampling is performed at the time of excisional biopsy.
3. The failure to recognize small, easily overlooked foci of invasive lobular carcinoma.

These differential diagnostic possibilities need to be consciously considered when interpreting needle biopsies of breast lesions *(18,19)*. If there are any reservations, then a definitive diagnosis should not be made and excisional biopsy should be recommended. When *in situ* carcinoma is diagnosed on needle biopsy, excisional biopsy should be performed because there may be invasive carcinoma as well. Biopsy is also recommended when ADH is diagnosed on needle biopsy, because there may be associated DCIS or invasive carcinoma *(20,21)*. This is particularly important if image guidance is not used. A study comparing the accuracy rates of breast biopsy techniques found that cutting needle biopsy without image guidance had a sensitivity of only 85%. This was considerably less than open breast biopsy (99%), FNA (96%), or cutting needle biopsy with image guidance (98%) *(22)*.

CONCLUSION

Claims involving breast cancer are frequent and are less likely to be successfully defended than most other malpractice cases. Most women present with no signs or symptoms other than the breast mass itself. It is the patient, not the doctor, who usually finds a lump, and these cases bring higher average indemnities.

Although these claims can involve physicians of any specialty, radiologists, pathologists and obstetrician/gynecologists are the most frequently targeted.

Mammography is often at the center of breast cancer claims. Surprisingly, the problem is more likely to be a communication error resulting from failure to take appropriate action following a correctly read study than it is to be an interpretation error.

One promising technique, computer-aided detection (CAD), offers the promise of reducing interpretation error and is just becoming more widely available. Mammogram films are taken in the usual manner and then scanned into a CAD system. The CAD system digitizes the mammogram and analyzes it for regions of interest, either clustered bright spots suggestive of microcalcification or dense regions suggesting a mass or architectural distortion. The radiologist first reads the film mammogram, then reviews the areas detected by the CAD system and evaluates them for clinical relevance. Published studies using blinded review of a prior "normal" mammogram in patients with newly diagnosed breast cancer showed that 23% of these films were, in fact, actionable. The CAD system detected 90% of these abnormal findings. This 20% increase in the breast cancer detection rate is impressive and, if CAD is widely adopted, may reduce the frequency of breast cancer malpractice claims *(23,24)*.

Many breast cancer claims are preventable. In cases where medical care has been suboptimal, the errors are usually obvious and most involve a short-circuiting of the diagnostic process or poor communication among physicians or between doctor and patient.

The following box contains a list of many pathways that lead to breast cancer litigation *(25)*:

1. Assuming that a mass in a young woman is not cancer.
2. Ignoring a breast mass in a pregnant or lactating woman.
3. Allowing a negative physical examination to delay biopsy in a patient with a suspicious mammogram.
4. Believing that the absence of "grave signs" of cancer is evidence against the presence of breast cancer.
5. Failure to document the history, physical examination findings, and a plan for follow-up.
6. Failure to order a diagnostic study, or order one but fail to assure it is completed.
7. Allowing a patient with a known lesion to be lost to follow-up.
8. Telling a patient not to worry about a mass she brings to your attention.
9. Failure to suggest breast cancer screening in appropriate patients.
10. Failure to assure that breast cancer screening includes both a physical examination and a mammogram.
11. Failure to discuss breast cancer prevention in high-risk patients.
12. Failure to advise family screening for a patient with a strong family history of breast cancer or who is known to carry Breast Cancer 1/2 genes.
13. Dismissing palpable axillary lymph nodes as simply "normal."
14. Telling a patient that she would have been cured "if only we had found the lesion earlier."
15. Allowing a negative or indeterminate mammogram to delay biopsy of a breast mass.
16. Allowing a negative breast ultrasound to exclude cancer in the face of an indeterminate mammogram.
17. Reading a technically unsatisfactory mammogram.
18. Failure to compare a current mammogram to prior studies.
19. Failure to inform the referring physician of suspicious findings.
20. Filing an abnormal mammogram report without informing the patient.
21. Performing a mammogram on a self-referred patient without arranging for clinical follow-up.
22. Telling a patient that with the benefit of hindsight, a nonspecific finding on a prior mammogram was actually cancer.
23. Issuing a pathology report without reviewing prior biopsies.
24. Failure to do specimen mammography on a biopsy performed for evaluation of a mammographic abnormality.

25. Allowing a negative FNA of a palpable mass to exclude a diagnosis of breast cancer.
26. Performing definitive breast surgery relying on an outside pathology report from a pathologist that you do not know.
27. Performing definitive breast surgery without waiting for the final pathology report on a biopsy or FNA.
28. Failure to offer breast conservation therapy to appropriate patients.
29. Treating enlarged axillary lymph nodes with antibiotics without assuring complete resolution.
30. Assuming a patient will be grateful because your decision to delay biopsy of a lesion, which proved to be malignant, was based on sound clinical judgment.

Each of these 30 ways of getting sued for breast cancer has, in fact, produced litigation. The last one is particularly troublesome, because it says our system does not reward even the responsible exercise of clinical judgment unless the outcome is perfect. No physician believes good clinical practice is possible without good clinical judgment, and none wants to practice purely defensive medicine. Nonetheless, in the current medical-legal environment, anything other than the earliest possible diagnosis of breast cancer may produce a malpractice claim.

REFERENCES

1. Anderson R. Breast cancer lawsuits. The Doctors Advocate 2001; Second Quarter:1.
2. Anderson R. Breast cancer lawsuit outcomes. The Doctors Advocate 2002; First Quarter:1.
3. Anderson R. Breast cancer lawsuit outcomes, part II. The Doctors Advocate 2002; Second Quarter:1.
4. Anderson R. Breast cancer study conclusions. The Doctors Advocate 2002; Third Quarter:1.
5. The Doctors Company data on file. Napa, CA 2002.
5a. Kerlkowske K, Grady D, Barclay J, et al. Likelihood ratios for modern screening mammography. JAMA 1996;276(1):39–43.
6. Beam CA, Layde PM, Sullivan DC. Variability in the interpretation of screening mammograms by US radiologists. Arch Intern Med 1996;156(2):209–213.
7. Troxel DB. Breast biopsy and fine needle aspiration. The Doctors Advocate 2002; Third Quarter:2–10.
8. Troxel DB. Diagnostic errors in surgical pathology uncovered by a review of malpractice claims. Int J Surg Pathol 2000;8:335–337.
9. Troxel DB. Malpractice claims involving breast pathology. Pathol Case Reviews 1999; 4:224–228.
10. Layfield LJ, Mooney EE, Glasgow B, et al. What constitutes an adequate smear in fine-needle aspiration cytology of the breast? Cancer (Cancer Cytopathology) 1997;81:16–21.

11. Boerner S, Sneige N. Specimen adequacy and false negative diagnosis rate in fine-needle aspirates of palpable breast masses. Cancer (Cancer Cytopathology) 1998; 84:344–348.

12. Abele J, Stanley MW, Miller TR, et al. What constitutes an adequate smear in fine needle aspiration cytology of the breast? Cancer (Cancer Cytopathology) 1998;84:57–61.

13. Jacobs T, Pliss N, Kouria G, et al. Carcinomas *in situ* of the breast with indeterminate features. Am J Surg Pathol 2001;25:229–236.

14. Maluf H, Swanson P, Koerner C. Solid low-grade *in situ* carcinoma of the breast. Am J Surg Pathol 2001;25:237–244.

15. Schnitt S, Connolly L, Tavassoli F, et al. Interobserver reproducibility in the diagnosis of ductal proliferative lesions using standardized criteria. Am J Surg Pathol 1992;16:1133–1143.

16. Palazzo J, Hyslop BS. Hyperplastic ductal and lobular lesions and carcinomas *in situ* of the breast: reproducibility of current diagnostic criteria among community- and academic-based pathologists. Breast J 1998;4:230–237.

17. Wells W, Carney P, Eliassen M, Grove M, Tosteson A. Pathololgists agreement with experts and reproducibility of breast ductal carcinoma-*in-situ* classification schemes. Am J Surg Pathol 2000;24:651–659.

18. Hoda S, Rosen P. Practical considertions in the pathologic diagnosis of needle core biopsies of breast. Am J Clin Pathol 2002;118:101–108.

19. Jacobs T, Connolly J, Schnitt S. Nonmalignant lesions in breast core needle biopsies. Am J Surg Pathol 2002;26(9):1095–1010.

20. Jackman R, Nowels K, Shepard M, et al. Stereotaxic large-core needle biopsy of 450 nonpalpable breast lesions with surgical correlation in lesions with cancer or atypical hyperplasia. Radiology 1994;193:91–95.

21. Renshaw A, Cartagena N, Schenkman R, et al. Atypical duct hyperplasia in breast core needle biopsies. Am J Clin Pathol 2001;116:92–96.

22. Antley C, Mooney E, Layfield L. A comparison of accuracy rates between open biopsy, cutting-needle biopsy, and fine-needle aspiration biopsy of the breast: a 3-year experience. Breast J 1998;4:3–8.

23. Burhenne LJW, Wood SA, D'Orsi CJ, et al. Potential contribution of computer-aided detection to the sensitivity of screening mammography. Radiology 2000; 215:554–562.

24. Chidley E. Assessing new mammography technologies. Radiology Today 2001;24.

25. Anderson R. Getting sued for breast cancer. The Doctors Advocate 2001; Third Quarter:1.

13 Pap Smear Litigation

David B. Troxel, MD, FCAP

SUMMARY

This chapter reviews The Doctors Company experience with medical liability claims involving the Pap smear. The historical factors leading to the explosive growth in Pap smear litigation are discussed and an expert medical panel's analysis of the sources of error in the Pap smear are presented in detail. The panel's recommendations for reducing the Pap smear's inherent false-negative rate, thereby decreasing patient injury from "missed" cervical cancers and their precursors, are reviewed. Finally, new technologies and strategies that enhance the Pap test's sensitivity (liquid-based cytology and DNA testing for human papillomavirus) are presented.

Key Words: Pap smear liability; Pap smear sensitivity; Pap smear false-negative rate; cervical cancer; human papillomavirus; liquid-based cytology.

INTRODUCTION

During the 1990s, both the frequency and severity (average indemnity paid per allocated claim) of claims involving cervical cytology (Pap smears) increased dramatically and became the most important source of malpractice liability for pathologists and pathology laboratories. The severity of pathology claims had become among the highest

From: *Medical Malpractice: A Physician's Sourcebook*
Edited by: R. E. Anderson © Humana Press Inc., Totowa, NJ

of all specialties—on a par with trauma surgery and obstetrics/gynecology (Ob/Gyn).

The Doctors Company (TDC) is a national physician-owned medical malpractice insurance company that covers more than 1200 pathologists. Table 1 documents its experience with Pap smear claims from 1992 to 2002.

Claims involving Pap smears showed alarming growth beginning in 1993. There were many reasons for this increase, including the landmark article published in November 1987 in the *Wall Street Journal* entitled "Lax Laboratories: The Pap Test Misses Much Cervical Cancer Through Labs Errors," which alerted the public to the fact that a Pap smear may be falsely negative. The article implied that false-negative Pap tests resulted largely from carelessness. This led to passage of the Clinical Laboratory Improvement Act of 1988 (CLIA 88) that legislated comprehensive regulation of the gynecologic cytology laboratory. Subsequently, there was extensive media coverage of women dying from cervical cancers that had been "missed" on prior Pap smears because of "laboratory error." A consequence of this publicity was that women diagnosed with cervical cancer, and their attorneys, would request that an "expert" review all prior "negative" Pap smears. This was reinforced by CLIA 88 that required review of all prior negative Pap smears in the 5 years preceeding a new diagnosis of a high-grade squamous intraepithelial lesion (HSIL) or carcinoma. Thus, a frequent scenario leading to a Pap smear claim involved a false-negative smear "discovered" upon review of prior "negatives" in a woman diagnosed with cervical carcinoma.

To put the potential magnitude of this problem in perspective, a study by the College of American Pathologists (CAP) of the 5-year "look back" at previous negative Pap smears following the diagnosis of HSIL/carcinoma found that 10% of prior smears were false-negatives for squamous intraepithelial lesion (SIL)/carcinoma *(1)*. If atypical squamous cells of undetermined significance (ASC-US) were included, 20% of prior smears were false-negatives. In 1996, the American Cancer Society predicted 15,700 new cases of cervical cancer and 4700 deaths. Published studies indicated that 60 to 75% of women dying from cervical cancer either never had a Pap smear or had not had one in the 5 years prior to diagnosis *(2,3)*. Therefore, if one assumed that 40% of the predicted new cases of cervical carcinoma had a single Pap smear in the prior 5 years with a 20% false-negative rate, there was a potential for 1256 new claims for failure to diagnose cervical carcinoma on a Pap smear in 1996 alone!

Table 1
Pap Smear/Cervical Cytology Claims, Includes Pathology and Lab Experience

Report Year	Allocated Claims	Case Incurred Indemnity	Case Incurred ALAE	Case Incurred Severity	% of Total Path/Lab Experience Claims	% of Total Path/Lab Experience Indemnity	% of Total Path/Lab Experience ALAE	Pathology Mature Exposures	Pathology Claims	Pathology Frequency (per 100 Docs)
1991 & Prior	66	4,219,200	1,395,335	85,069	13	17	18	1590	14	0.9
1992	14	203,000	156,377	25,670	10	3	7	1644	38	2.3
1993	41	2,633,749	380,180	73,510	23	20	14	1594	28	1.8
1994	31	706,749	523,487	39,685	18	8	21	1596	50	3.1
1995	52	6,444,200	744,033	138,235	29	47	32	1412	30	2.1
1996	30	4,963,067	1,129,457	203,084	19	39	28	1318	22	1.7
1997	23	319,875	376,849	30,292	19	4	19	1208	22	1.8
1998	26	8,911,875	917,966	378,071	26	62	41	1063	13	1.2
1999	14	2,879,000	420,153	235,654	18	43	21	920	8	0.9
2000	8	2,790,000	192,632	372,829	7	17	8	777	5	0.6
2001	7	2,247,500	96,717	334,888	10	23	9	796	15	1.9
2002	15	1,971,000	124,147	139,676	24	40	22			
Total	327	38,289,215	6,457,332	136,840	18	27	21	13,918	245	1.8

Data evaluated as of 5/31/03.

169

This potential magnitude of Pap smear liability focused the pathology community's attention on the need to better understand the causes of the false-negative Pap test and to develop strategies to deal with this problem. The difficulty was aggravated by the fact that Pap smears had long been a "loss leader" for large independent laboratories attempting to gain market share and was reimbursed well below cost by many health insurers, Medicare, and Medicaid. Combined with the deteriorating liability climate, this caused many laboratories to consider no longer accepting Pap smears. At stake was the survival of the Pap smear as an effective, affordable, widely available screening test for cervical cancer, as well as the future of cytology as a diagnostic discipline.

An additional concern was the effect managed care might have on Pap smear liability. Would the trend toward mandating lab test referral to large regional laboratories (their lower marginal costs associated with large Pap smear volumes helped to ameliorate poor reimbursement) interfere with pathologist–physician communication and follow-up cytologic/histologic correlation? Would the frequent patient change of plans and doctors interfere with appropriate Pap smear follow-up? What would the impact be of shifting the responsibility for collecting Pap smears and the appropriate follow-up of abnormal results from gynecologists to primary care physicians? Would the frequency of the annual screening Pap smear be reduced by the pressures of cost containment and diminish the opportunity to detect lesions "missed" on prior false-negative Pap smears?

At TDC, physician consultants and panels of medical experts periodically meet to review claims from each medical specialty as part of malpractice risk management and loss prevention. In an attempt to manage the escalating frequency of Pap smear claims, a panel composed of cytology experts and gynecologists met in 1996 to discuss liability issues involving cervical cytology. The panels' written recommendations (4) were distributed to all insured pathologists, gynecologists, and primary care physicians and presented at state and national professional society meetings.

LIMITING PAP SMEAR LIABILITY: PANEL RECOMMENDATIONS

An Annual Pap Smear is Important

An ideal screening test is one that is always abnormal in the presence of disease, that is, it has a sensitivity of 100%. False-positive results are acceptable and are detected by subsequent specific (and expensive) testing. False-negatives are undesirable because patients with disease will be missed. As a screening test for cervical cancer detection, the Pap smear is largely responsible for the 70% decline in deaths from cervical cancer that has occurred over the past 50 years (from 30 to 2.6 cases per 100,000 population). Yet, ironically, the Pap smear falls far short of the ideal 100% sensitivity of a screening test. Although there is a wide range in the reported false-negative rate for a single conventional Pap smear, 15–25% is widely accepted (including both sampling and laboratory false-negatives). A 20–30% false-negative rate has been reported for biopsy-proven HSIL/cancer when Pap tests showing at least ASC-US are considered positive *(5)*. Sampling false-negatives (absence of abnormal cells on the smear) are slightly more common than laboratory false-negatives, which are divided about evenly between screening errors made by cytotechnologists and interpretation errors made by pathologists. Every laboratory has false-negatives—including the very best laboratories and those supervised by experts!

The low-grade squamous intraepithelial lesion (LSIL) accounts for most false-negative Pap smears, and about half of these lesions regress spontaneously. The remaining lesions persist or may progress. For those that progress, the evolution is usually slow; however, 20 to 30% of women with LSIL on Pap smear have HSIL on biopsy. Therefore, in 1996, the consequence of a false-negative was best minimized by obtaining a Pap smear annually (i.e., there are more opportunities to detect the lesion.) Thus, the most cost-effective way to manage the false-negative rate inherent in the conventional Pap smear, and to further reduce the incidence of cervical cancer, was to increase Pap smear frequency and keep its cost low.

Sources of Error for the Pap Smear
SAMPLING ERRORS

Sampling errors account for 50–60% of false-negatives in which abnormal cells are not present on the smear either because they were not present in the collected sample or they were present but not recovered when the smear was prepared. Liquid-based cytology techniques enhance the recovery of abnormal cells collected in the cervical sample, and with reported false-negative rates of 5–15% *(5,6)*, they are more sensitive than the conventional Pap smear in detecting SILs.

SCREENING ERRORS

Screening errors account for about one-half of laboratory false-negatives and result from two major causes.

Failure to Detect Abnormal Cells Present on the Smear

The following are reasons for the failure to detect abnormal cells on a smear:

1. Smears may have too few cells; 100 abnormal cells per smear seems to be a minimum threshold for recognition by the screening cytotechnologist.
2. Smears may show small single cells called "no-see-ums." These are present in some cases of HSILs. They are small cells (<15 micra) with a high nuclear/cytoplasmic ratio, minimal chromatin abnormalities, and irregular nuclear membranes ("raisinoid" nuclei). The large cells with low nuclear/cytoplasmic ratios and "ugly" nuclei seen in LSILs are less frequently missed.
3. Hyperchromatic crowded groups of cells are often difficult to accurately classify. They may be normal endometrial cells or benign basal cells seen in atrophy, but abnormal cells from HSILs can also mimic this appearance.
4. "Litigation" cells can look like virtually anything, especially in retrospect (7).

In 1996, new technologies and techniques were emerging that were designed to improve recognition of missed cells, increase the sensitivity of the Pap smear, and reduce false-negatives. These included liquid-based cytology, automated processing and screening, automated and manual rescreening of both negative Pap smears and smears showing ASC-US, and rapid rescreening. However, these techniques were expensive, and because the increased costs were not offset by higher reimbursement, few laboratories were able to provide them. Some pathologists expressed concern that even if reimbursed, the higher cost may reduce both access to the Pap smear and its frequency, whereas others wondered if a higher "community standard" for the frequency of false-negative Pap smears would increase the public's expectation of perfection and thereby increase liability.

Failure to Recognize Unsatisfactory Pap Smears

CLIA 88 prohibits making a diagnosis of "negative for intraepithelial lesion or malignancy" on an unsatisfactory Pap smear. However, a Pap smear with abnormal epithelial cells must never be interpreted as "unsatisfactory for evaluation." For this reason, potentially unsatisfactory smears must be very carefully screened for the presence of abnormal cells before reporting them as unsatisfactory. The fact that CLIA 88 prohibits making a diagnosis on unsatisfactory Pap smears assures liability if a woman with cervical cancer had a prior Pap smear diagnosed as "negative for intraepithelial lesion or malignancy" that on retrospective review is found to be unsatisfactory. For these reasons, every laboratory should have written policies defining specimen adequacy; today these should be based on the 2001 Bethesda System recommendations. These criteria include the presence of at least 10 well-preserved endocervical or squamous metaplastic cells and 8000–12,000 squamous cells (5000 for liquid-based preparations) *(8)*. For computerized labs, "edits" should be created to assure that diagnoses are not assigned to unsatisfactory smears.

INTERPRETATION ERRORS

Interpretation errors account for the other 50% of laboratory false-negatives. Some of the causes of interpretation errors are listed here:

1. ASC-US is a poorly defined diagnostic category and represents the pathologist's interpretative "gray zone." Diagnostic criteria are not uniformly agreed on and there is poor inter- and intraobserver reproducibility *(9,10)*. Expert members of the CAP Cytopathology Committee reached 80% consensus on the diagnosis of ASC-US on only 20% of cases reviewed; there was not 100% consensus on any case. Approximately 2 million Pap tests in the United States are diagnosed as ASC-US each year. Therefore, finding ASC-US on retrospective review of a "negative" Pap smear should never be the sole basis for judging a false-negative Pap smear to be below the standard of practice. However, because about 26% of women with ASC-US are subsequently diagnosed with SILs (up to one in four as HSILs), rescreening of all ASC-US cases is recommended as a quality assurance (QA) procedure. Furthermore, when atypical cells are found on a Pap smear, it is important that they not be characterized with terms such as "non-neoplastic" or "benign." This may be interpreted by the clinician to mean that a repeat Pap smear or appropriate follow-up study is not necessary. Use of the 2001 Bethesda System terminology *(8)* is an appropriate way to deal with this situation (i.e., "Atypical Squamous Cells of Undetermined Significance [ASC-US]"), coupled with a recommendation for appropriate follow-up studies.

2. Misinterpretation of an "epithelial cell abnormality" as "negative for intraepithelial lesion or malignancy," (e.g., cervical adenocarcinoma cells misinterpreted as reactive endocervical cells).

3. Failure to look carefully for abnormal cells in the "neighborhood" of parakeratotic cells. Because abnormal cells tend to occur in linear streaks, pathologists must look carefully at screened smears with lines of dots or look to either side of dotted abnormal cells for other abnormal cells.

Recommended Strategies for Alerting Physicians
to the Pap Smear's Inherent False-Negative Rate

The following are recommended strategies for alerting physicians to the Pap smear's inherent false-negative rate:

1. Include a "statement" in the Pap smear report reminding the clinician (and patient) that the Pap smear is a screening test with an irreducible false-negative rate, the consequences of which can be minimized by obtaining an annual Pap smear. It is important to educate the public, primary care physicians, and gynecologists about the limitations of the Pap smear so that they have realistic expectations about its sensitivity and understand why it is important to obtain a Pap smear annually.

2. Provide the referring physician with patient information cards explaining in easy to understand lay terms that although the conventional Pap smear's accuracy in detecting abnormalities is about 70–80%, it is not perfect, and, therefore, an annual Pap smear is important. The patient may be asked to sign the card to indicate that it has been read. (TDC sent such a poster containing this information to its insured physicians in 1999.)

3. Encourage annual Pap smears. Monthly or quarterly, labs should send each physician a list of their patients who had negative Pap smears in the same month or quarter of the prior year, reminding the physician to obtain a repeat "annual" Pap smear.

Legal and Regulatory Considerations
Affecting Pap Smear Liability

The following are legal and regulatory considerations affecting Pap smear liability:

1. CLIA 88 requires a 5-year "look back" at prior negatives when a Pap smear shows HSILs or carcinoma. An amended report must be issued and the referring physician notified if a changed diagnosis would affect patient care. "Would affect patient care," means at the current time (Health Care Financing Administration's interpretation), not at the time of the original diagnosis. Therefore, issue an amended report only if it affects current patient care, and issue it under the current accession number and not under the original accession number. This will ensure that the physician currently responsible for managing the patient's care is informed. Also, although one should rescreen the prior negatives thoroughly, avoid speculative interpretation of questionable findings (e.g., ASC-US).

2. CLIA 88 mandated QA and quality control (QC) records, including the 5-year "look back" at prior negatives, may be admissible in court

depending on whether or not the court interprets them as being protected by state peer-review laws. Therefore, it is important to label all such records as QA or QC and file them separately from other lab records.

3. Make cytologic-histologic correlation statements in the report only if it affects patient care. Otherwise, it is preferable to make these correlations in your QA records and only for biopsies collected within 60 to 100 days of the abnormal Pap smear. Because many lesions regress, there is often poor correlation after 100 days.

4. Although false-positive Pap smears increase health care costs, they seldom incur legal liability and infrequently result in lawsuits. Remember, the Pap smear is a screening test (not a definitive diagnostic test), and lowering the threshold for diagnosing an abnormality increases its sensitivity.

5. When asked by an attorney to provide "expert" review of a Pap smear, the reviewer should ask, "How would this smear have been read by a competent cytologist in the usual practice environment?" Preferably, the Pap smear in question should be subjected to blinded rescreening by a panel of experienced cytologists (who are not necessarily experts) and as one of a larger number of both normal and abnormal slides, without knowledge of the clinical outcome or alleged error *(11)*. Too often, reviewers focus on a few cells that in retrospect could be interpreted as ASC-US and conclude, "These should not have been missed," adding that, "If noted, follow-up may have detected the missed cancer." This is particularly troublesome because criteria for recognizing atypical squamous cells are not well-defined and both inter- and intraobserver reproducibility in diagnosing ASC-US is low.

6. Discard slides upon completion of the required retention period. Both CLIA 88 standards and the CAP laboratory accreditation program standards require the retention of cytology slides (both normal and abnormal) for 5 years. Some states may have different requirements.

Issues Often Raised in Court

The following are some issues that may be raised in litigation involving Pap smears:

1 Failure to adhere to current CLIA 88 regulations and/or to follow practices recommended by professional societies. This may include screening Pap smears in locations other than the laboratory premises or violating workload standards. Workload standard violations may include:

a. Piecework with payment "by the slide."

b. "Piggyback jobs"—one full-time and another part-time.

c. Failure to document the number of slides screened and the number of hours spent screening in a 24-hour period.

2. Failure to participate in interlaboratory comparison or proficiency testing programs, such as the CAP PAP program. Although there are no data to demonstrate that participation in an external proficiency testing program lessens a laboratory's liability, participation is encouraged for its educational and QA value.
3. Failure to recognize that a Pap smear is "unsatisfactory for evaluation."
4. Failure to use the current Bethesda System terminology *(8)*, which is now part of the cytology standard of practice. Do not use an obsolete "class" reporting system.

Preventative Measures

The followiwng list contains some preventative measures that can be taken:

1. Have a clearly defined and written QA program. Implement the program, document it, and take QA procedures seriously.
2. Comply with CLIA 88 and state regulatory requirements. Pathologists must make certain that their laboratories adhere to current CLIA 88 standards, because they have become part of the legal definition of the standard of care.
3. Establish a cytology slide-release procedure *(12)*. Cytology slides are not replaceable if lost or broken. Therefore, in the absence of a subpoena, do not send cytology slides to an attorney for review. Instead, require the plaintiff's "experts" to come to your lab to review the slides under your direct supervision. If you receive a subpoena, notify your malpractice insurer. Submit original slides only if so ordered by the court.
4. Have and follow written cytology policies and procedures.
5. Evaluate and report the adequacy of each specimen, utilizing the Bethesda System specimen adequacy criteria.
6. Provide recommendations for follow-up of Pap smears with epithelial cell abnormalities or specimen adequacy limitations, especially for nongynecologists. The 2001 Consensus Guidelines for Cervical Cytological Abnormalities sponsored by the American Society for Colposcopy and Cervical Pathology (ASCCP) are recommended *(13)*.
7. Use outside expert consultation for problem Pap smears, when appropriate.
8. Restrict discussions about potential claims to individuals within your practice group. Limit the number of people within your group who review a potential problem Pap smear, because anyone who reviews it may be subsequently deposed.
9. Notify your insurance company early if you suspect that a claim may be filed.

Long-Term Solutions and Questions to Explore

Long-term solutions and questions that should be explored include the following:

1. Define a new standard of care for the Pap smear. The zero-error standard is not attainable. We need a reasonable practitioner standard or a process standard, not an outcome standard; following the procedures proven to minimize the false-negative rate (complying with CLIA 88 regulations is a minimum standard) should become the standard of care rather than the current unattainable standard of having a zero false-negative rate.

2. Develop criteria that define an expert witness and create a national registry of certified expert witnesses.

3. Identify how to effectively respond to misleading testimony given by a plaintiff's "expert" witness. The Guidelines for Review of PAP Smears in the Context of Litigation or Potential Litigation (a state and national professional society-endorsed process for objective slide review) are recommended *(11)*.

4. Facilitate the use of blinded expert review panels *(11)*.

5. Determine if pathologists who are board certified in cytopathology are less apt to make interpretative errors than general pathologists, less apt to experience liability claims when errors are made, and are easier to defend when a claim is filed.

6. Determine if laboratories with low volumes (<5000–10,000 Pap smears per year) and laboratories without cytotechnologists (where the screening is done by a pathologist) are at a higher risk of malpractice. The results of a CAP Interlaboratory Comparison Program in Cervical Cytology published in 1993 concluded that pathologist false-negative and false-positive rates and technologist false-negative rates were lower in laboratories processing more than 20,000 Pap smears each year, compared with labs processing less than 10,000 Pap smears each year *(14)*.

CONCLUSION

These recommendations were distributed in 1997. Beginning in 1999, there appears to have been a decrease in frequency of Pap smear claims— unfortunately offset by an increase in claims severity. Because risk management can only affect frequency, whereas severity is a reflection of societal values and our legal system, it is tempting to speculate that these recommendations, coupled with the efforts of professional societies also attempting to identify sources of error in the Pap smear *(15)*, were in some measure effective.

Fortunately, 7 years after this risk-management guideline was published, new diagnostic strategies have emerged to detect cervical cancer and its precursor lesions. These strategies have greater sensitivity than the conventional Pap smear with correspondingly lower false-negative rates. Most are based on our understanding that human papillomavirus (HPV) infection is the underlying cause of cervical cancer and its precursors. Carcinogenic high-risk HPV types can be identified in liquid-based cytology specimens or in specimens obtained subsequent to collecting a conventional Pap smear.

The National Cancer Institute's ASC-US/LSIL Triage Study (ALTS; *16*) involved 3488 women with ASC-US and 1572 with LSIL and evaluated three alternative methods of management: immediate colposcopy, cytologic follow-up, and triage by HPV DNA testing (for 13 oncogenic HPV types utilizing liquid-based cytology). These women were followed for 2 years. The conclusions of the study were as follows:

1. In women with a diagnosis of ASC-US, HPV DNA testing is as sensitive as colposcopy in detecting HSIL/carcinoma, particularly in women older than age 29 years. When ASC-US is diagnosed, automatically testing for HPV permits triaging those who are HPV-positive to colposcopy (55%), whereas those who are HPV-negative can be followed with a repeat Pap test in 12 months (45%).
2. Reflex HPV testing is not an effective triage method for LSILs because of the high prevalence of high-risk HPV types. Most women with LSILs should be referred for colposcopic examination, although management options may differ for adolescent, pregnant, and postmenopausal women.
3. Both HPV-positive patients with ASC-US and LSIL can be followed after colposcopy with 12-month HPV testing. Their risk of developing HSIL is approx 26% at 2 years.
4. HPV testing also shows promise as a primary screening test, because its sensitivity exceeds that of cytology. However, its specificity is somewhat lower, especially in women younger than age 30 years.
5. HPV DNA testing combined with a cytology test ("DNA with Pap" Test) is now approved by the Food and Drug Administration for women age 30 years and older. Its sensitivity for detecting HSIL/carcinoma approaches 100% and has the potential to eliminate screening false-negatives, thereby decreasing risk for both patients and laboratories *(17)* .

These ALTS conclusions were the basis for the Consensus Guidelines for the Management of Women With Cervical Cytological Abnormalities developed by the ASCCP *(14)* . Pathologists and clinicians should become familiar with these guidelines, and pathologists should consider making follow-up recommendations in their Pap reports. For liquid-based cytology ASC-US cases, a recommendation such as "consider immediate HPV DNA testing, diagnostic colposcopy, or a repeat Pap test in 4 to 6 months" may be appropriate.

Over the past 7 years, there has been an increase in the proportion of cervical cancers that are adenocarcinomas (approx one in three). The conventional Pap test is not effective in detecting cervical adenocarcinoma; the abnormal cells are often interpreted as "atypical glandular cells of undetermined significance" or "reactive endocervical cells." HPV DNA testing shows promise in detecting a high percentage of these cases as well.

Finally, the American Cancer Society revised its cervical cancer screening guidelines in 2002 as follows:

* Screening should begin 3 years after becoming sexually active but no later than 21 years of age.
* A conventional Pap test should be done annually, or a liquid-based cytology test should be obtained every 2 years until age 30 years.
* If there have been three consecutive negative cytology tests, then screening should continue every 2 to 3 years thereafter.

REFERENCES

1. Jones B. Rescreening in gynecologic cytology. Arch Pathol Lab Med 1995;119: 1097–1103.
2. Janerich D, Hadjimichael O, Schwartz PE, et al. The screening histories of women with invasive cervical cancer in Connecticut. Am J Pub Health 1995; 85: 791–794.
3. NCI Consensus Conference, April 1996.
4. Troxel D. Risk Management Guidelines for Cervical Cytology. The Doctors Company, 1997.
5. Claver C, Masure M, Bory J-P, et al. Human papillomavirus testing in primary screening for the detection of high grade cervical lesions. Br J Cancer 2001;89: 1616–1623.
6. Davey D, Zarbo R. Introduction and commentary, strategic science symposium on human papillomavirus testing. Arch Pathol Lab Med 2003;127:927–929.
7. Frable W. Litigation cells: definition and observations on a cell type in cervical vaginal smears not addressed by the Bethesda system. Diagn Cytopathol 1994;11: 213–215.
8. The 2001 Bethesda System, consensus statement, terminology for reporting results of cervical cytology. JAMA 2002;287:2114–2118.
9. Bonfiglio T. Atypical squamous of undetermined significance: a continuing controversy. Cancer (cytopathol) 2002;96:125–127.
10. Boerner S, Katz R. On the origins of "atypical squamous cells of undetermined significance": the evolution of a diagnostic term. Advances in Anatomic Path 1997;4:221–231.

11. Fitzgibbons P, Austin M. Expert review of histologic slides and Papanicolaou tests in the context of litigation or potential litigation. Arch Pathol Lab Med 2000; 124:1717–1719.
12. "Requests for Pathology Specimens"—a TDC Risk Management Guideline.
13. Wright T, Cox J, Massad L, et al. 2001 Consensus Guidelines for the Management of Women With Cervical Cytological Abnormalities. JAMA 2002;287:2120–2137.
14. Davey D, Nielsen M, Frable W, et al. Improving accuracy in gynecologic cytology. Arch Pathol Lab Med 1993;117:1193–1198.
15. June 1996 CAP Conference on "Liability and Quality Issues in Cervicovaginal Cytology," Seattle. The entire proceedings are published in Arch Pathol Lab Med 1997;121:205–342.
16. Schiffman M, Solomon D. Findings to date from the ASCUS-LSIL Triage Study (ALTS). Arch Pathol Lab Med 2003;127:946–949.
17. Lorincz A, Richart R. Human Papillomavirus DNA testing as an adjunct to cytology in cervical screening programs. Arch Pathol Lab Med 2003;127:959–967.

14 Medical Liability in Plastic and Reconstructive Surgery

Mark Gorney, MD

SUMMARY

The great majority of claims against plastic surgeons are concentrated in less than 10 procedures, all of them elective or aesthetic. Because the patient is the ultimate judge of satisfaction in the outcome, there is a greater burden of responsibility on the surgeon for patient selection, preoperative disclosure, and documentation. The essential elements of each are reviewed, as are the current standards of care for the specialty.

Key Words: Warranty; informed consent; hypertrophic scar; body dysmorphic syndrome; therapeutic alliance.

LEGAL PRINCIPLES APPLIED TO PLASTIC SURGERY

Standard of Care

Malpractice generally means treatment that is contrary to accepted medical standards and that produces injurious results in the patient. Most medical malpractice actions are based on laws governing negligence. Thus, the cause of action is usually the failure of the physician to exercise that reasonable degree of skill, learning, and care ordinarily possessed by others of the same profession in the community. Whereas in the past, the term community was accepted geographically, it is now based on the supposition that all doctors keep up with the latest devel-

From: *Medical Malpractice: A Physician's Sourcebook*
Edited by: R. E. Anderson © Humana Press Inc., Totowa, NJ

opments in their field. Today, community is generally interpreted as a "specialty community." The standards are now those of the specialty as a whole without regard to geographic location. This series of norms is commonly referred to as "standard of care."

Warranty

The law holds that by merely engaging to render treatment, a doctor warrants that he or she has the learning and skill of the average member of that specialty and that he or she will apply that learning and skill with ordinary and reasonable care. The warranty is one of due care. It is legally implied. It need not be mentioned by the physician or the patient. However, the warranty is one of service, not cure. Thus, the doctor does not imply that the operation will be a success, that results will be favorable, or that he or she will not commit any medical errors not caused by lack of skill or care.

Disclosure

While attempting to define the yardstick of disclosure, the courts divide medical and surgical procedures into two categories:

1. Common procedures that incur minor or remote serious risk (e.g., the administration of acetaminophen).
2. Procedures involving serious risks that the doctor has an affirmative duty to disclose. He or she is bound to explain in detail the complications that might possibly occur.

Affirmative duty means that the physician is obliged to disclose risks on his or her own, without waiting for the patient to ask. The courts have long held that it is the patient, not the physician, who has the prerogative of determining what is in his or her best interests. Thus, the surgeon is legally obligated to discuss with the patient therapeutic alternatives and their particular hazards to provide sufficient information to determine the individual's own best interest. The extent of explanation the detail are dictated by a balance between the surgeon's judgments about his or her patient and the legal requirements applicable. It is simply not possible to tell patients everything without unnecessarily dissuading them from appropriate treatment. Rather, the law holds that patients must be told the most probable of known dangers and the percentage likelihood. More remote risks may be disclosed in general terms, while placing them in a context of suffering from any unusual event.

Obviously, the most common complications should be volunteered frankly and openly, and their probability, based on the surgeon's personal experience, should also be discussed. Finally, any or all of this information is wasted unless it is documented in the patient's record. For legal purposes, if it is not in the record, it never happened.

Informing Your Patients Before They Consent

In the last 5 years, most medical liability carriers have experienced a significant increase in claims alleging failure to obtain a proper informed consent prior to treatment. This trend is particularly noticeable in claims against surgical specialties performing elective procedures.

Informed consent means that adult patients who are capable of rational communication must be provided with sufficient information about risks, benefits, and alternatives to make an informed decision regarding a proposed course of treatment. (The same is true for emancipated or self-sufficient minor patients.) In most states, physicians have an affirmative duty to disclose such information. This means that you must not wait for questions from your patients; you must volunteer the information.

Without informed consent, you risk legal liability for a complication or untoward result, even if it was not caused negligently.

The essence of this widely accepted legal doctrine is that patient must be given all information about risks that are relevant to a meaningful decision-making process. It is the prerogative of the patient, not the physician, to determine the direction in which it is believed that his or her best interests lie. Thus, reasonable familiarity with therapeutic and/ or diagnostic alternatives and their hazards is essential.

Do patients have the legal right to make bad judgments because they fear a possible complication? Increasingly, the courts answer affirmatively. Once the information has been fully disclosed, that aspect of the physician's obligation has been fulfilled. The final decision on therapy usually rests with the patient.

"Prudent Patient" Test

In many states, the most important element in claims involving disputes over informed consent is the prudent patient test. The judge will inform the jury that there is no liability on the doctor's part if a prudent person in the patient's position would have accepted the treatment had he or she been adequately informed of all significant perils. Although this concept is subject to re-evaluation in hindsight, the prudent patient test becomes most meaningful where treatment is lifesaving or urgent.

The concept also may apply to simple procedures where the danger is commonly appreciated to be remote. In such cases, disclosure need not be extensive, and the prudent patient test will usually prevail.

Refusals

As part of medical counseling, many state laws mandate that physicians warn patients of the consequences involved with failing to heed medical advice by refusing treatment or diagnostic tests. Obviously, patients have a right to refuse. In such circumstances, it is essential that you carefully document such refusals and their consequences and that you verify and note that the patient understood the consequences.

Documentation is particularly important in cases involving malignancy, where rejection of tests may impair diagnosis and refusal of treatment may lead to a fatal outcome. Remember to date all such entries in the patient record.

If the information you present includes percentages or other specific figures that allow the patient to compare risks, then be certain that your figures conform to the latest reliable data.

Consent-in-Fact and Implied Consent

What is the distinction between ordinary consent to treatment (consent-in-fact) and informed consent? Simply stated, the latter verifies that the patient is aware of anticipated benefits, as well as risks and alternatives to a given procedure, treatment, or test. On the other hand, proceeding with treatment of any kind without actual consent is "unlawful touching" and, therefore, may be considered battery.

When the patient is unable to communicate rationally, as in many emergency cases, there may be a legally implied consent to treat. The implied consent in an emergency is assumed only for the duration of that emergency.

Minors

Except in urgent situations, treating minors without consent from a parent, legal guardian, appropriate government agency, or court carries a high risk of civil or even criminal charges. There are statutory exceptions, such as for an emancipated adolescent or a married minor. If you regularly treat young people, you should familiarize yourself with the existing statutory provisions in your state and keep up to date.

Religious and Other Obstacles

Occasionally, you may be placed in the difficult position of being refused permission to treat or conduct diagnostic tests on the basis of a patient's religious or other beliefs. Although grave consequences may ensue, there is little that you can do in most states beyond making an intense effort to convince the patient. In some states, court intervention may be obtained. Here too, knowing the law of the state in which you practice is advisable. In all cases, the informed refusal must be carefully documented.

If a patient is either a minor or incompetent (and the parent or guardian refuses treatment), and you know serious consequences will ensue if appropriate tests and/or treatment are not undertaken, then your legal and moral obligations change. You must then resort to a court order or another appropriate governmental process in an attempt to secure surrogate consent. The participation of personal or hospital legal counsel is advisable to ensure that the legal requirements applicable in your locale are met.

The Six Elements of Informed Consent

Where treatment is urgent (e.g., in a case of severe trauma), it may be needless and cruel to engage in extensive disclosure that could augment existing anxieties. However, you should inform the patient of the treatment's risks and consequences and record such discussions.

In general, it is important to discuss the following six elements of a valid informed consent with your patients and/or their families.

1. The diagnosis or suspected diagnosis.
2. The nature and purpose of the proposed treatment or procedure and its anticipated benefits.
3. The risks, complications, or side effects.
4. The probability of success, based on the patient's condition.
5. Reasonable available alternatives.
6. Possible consequences if advice is not followed.

In situations where the nature of the tests or treatment is purely elective, as with cosmetic surgery, the disclosure of risks and consequences may need to be expanded. Office literature can provide additional details about the procedure. In addition, an expanded discussion should take place regarding the foreseeable risks, possible untoward consequences, or unpleasant side effects associated with the procedure. This expansion is particularly necessary if the procedure is new, experimental, especially hazardous, purely for cosmetic purposes, or capable of altering sexual capacity or fertility.

Documentation

Written verification of consent to diagnostic or therapeutic procedures is crucial. However, also remember that in an increasing number of circumstances, laws now require the completion of specifically designed consent forms.

Studies indicate that physicians sometimes underestimate the patient's ability to understand. If your records disclose no discussion or consent, then the burden will be on you to demonstrate legally sufficient reasons for such absence.

It is a test of your good judgment of what to say to your patient and of how to say it to obtain meaningful consent without frightening the patient.

No permit or form will absolve you from responsibility if there is negligence, nor can a form guarantee that you will not be sued. Permits may vary from simple to incomprehensibly detailed. Most medical-legal authorities agree that a middle ground exists.

A well-drafted informed consent document is proof that you tried to give the patient sufficient information on which to base an intelligent decision. Such a document, supported by a handwritten note and entered in the patient's medical record, is often the key to a successful malpractice defense when the issue of consent to treatment arises.

The Therapeutic Alliance

Obtaining informed consent need not be an impersonal legal requirement. When properly conducted, the process of obtaining informed consent can help establish a "therapeutic alliance" and launch or reinforce a positive doctor–patient relationship. If an unfavorable outcome occurs, that relationship can be crucial to maintaining patient trust.

A common defense mechanism against uncertainty is for a patient to endow his or her doctor with omniscience in the science of medicine, an aura of omnipotence. By weighing how you say something as heavily as what you say, you can turn an anxiety-ridden ritual into an effective therapeutic alliance. Psychiatric literature refers to this as the sharing of uncertainty. Rather than shattering a patient's inherent trust in you by presenting an insensitive approach, your dialogue should be sympathetic to the patient's particular concerns or tensions and should project believable reactions to an anxious and difficult situation.

Consider, for example, the different effects that the following two statements would have:

1. "Here is a list of complications that could occur during your treatment [operation]. Please read the list and sign it."
2. "I wish I could guarantee you that there will be no problems during your treatment [operation], but that wouldn't be realistic. Sometimes there are problems that cannot be foreseen, and I want you to know about them. Please read about the possible problems, and let's talk about them."

By using the second statement, you can reduce the patient's omnipotent image of you to that of a more realistic and imperfect human being who is facing, and thus sharing, the same uncertainty. The implication is clear: we—you and I—are going to cooperate in doing something to your body that we hope will make you better, but you must assume some of the responsibility.

To allay anxiety, you may seek to reassure your patients. However, in so doing, be wary of creating unwarranted expectations or implying a guarantee.

Consider the different implications of these two statements:

1. "Don't worry about a thing. I've taken care of hundreds of cases like yours. You'll do just fine."
2. "Barring any unforeseen problems, I see no reason why you shouldn't do very well. I'll certainly do everything I can to help you."

If you make the first statement and the patient does not do "fine," he or she is likely to be angry with you. The second statement gently deflates the patient's fantasies to realistic proportions. This statement simultaneously reassures the patient and helps him or her to accept reality.

The therapeutic objective of informed consent should be to replace some of the patient's anxiety with a sense of his or her participation with you in the procedure. Such a sense of participation strengthens the therapeutic alliance between you and your patients. Instead of seeing each other as potential adversaries if an unfavorable or less-than-perfect outcome results, you and your patients are drawn closer by sharing acceptance and understanding of the uncertainty of clinical practice.

PATIENT-SELECTION CRITERIA

Contemporary plastic and reconstructive surgeons practicing in the United States will find it virtually impossible to end their careers unblemished by a claim of malpractice. However, well over half of these are preventable. Most are based either on failures of communication and patient-selection criteria, not on technical fault. Patient selection is an inexact science. It requires a mixture of surgical judgment and gut reaction. Regardless of technical ability, a surgeon who appears cold, arrogant, or insensitive is more likely to be sued than one who relates at a personal level. A surgeon who is warm, sensitive, and naturally caring, with a well-developed sense of humor and cordial attitude, is less likely to be the target of a malpractice claim.

Communication is the *sine qua non* of building a doctor–patient relationship. Unfortunately, the ability to communicate well is skill that cannot be learned easily in adulthood. It is an integral part of the surgeon's personality. However, there are a number of helpful guidelines.

Great Expectations

There are certain patients who have an unrealistic and idealized but vague conception of what elective aesthetic surgery is going to do for them. They anticipate a major change in lifestyle with immediate recognition of their newly acquired attractiveness. These patients have an unrealistic concept of where their surgical journey is taking them and have great difficulty in accepting the fact that any major surgical procedure carries inherent risk.

Excessively Demanding Patients

In general, the patient who brings photographs, drawings, and exact architectural specifications to the consultation should be managed with great caution. Such a patient has little comprehension that the surgeon is dealing with human flesh and blood, not wood or clay. This patient must be made to understand the realities of surgery, the vagaries of the healing process, and the margin of error that is a natural part of any elective procedure. Such patients show very little flexibility in accepting any failure on the part of the surgeon to deliver what was anticipated.

The Indecisive Patient

To the question "Doctor, do you think I ought to have this done?" the prudent surgeon should respond, "This is a decision that I cannot make for you. It is one you have to make yourself. I can tell you what I think we can achieve, but if you have any doubt whatsoever, I recommend strongly that you think about it carefully before deciding whether or not to accept the risks that I have discussed with you." The more the decision to undergo surgery is motivated from within and not "sold," the less likely recrimination will follow an unfavorable result.

The Immature Patient

The experienced surgeon should assess not only the physical but also the emotional maturity of the patient. The youthful or immature patient (age has no relationship to maturity) may have excessively romantic expectations and an unrealistic concept of what the surgery will achieve.

When confronted with the mirror postoperatively, they may react in disconcerting or even violent fashion if the degree of change achieved does not coincide with their preconceived notions.

The Secretive Patient

Certain patients wish to convert their surgery into a "secret" and request elaborate precautions to prevent anyone from knowing they are having cosmetic surgery. Aside from the fact that such arrangements are difficult to achieve, this tendency is a strong indication that the patient has a degree of guilt about the procedure. Thus, there is a higher likelihood of subsequent dissatisfaction.

Familial Disapproval

It is far more comfortable, although not essential, if the immediate family approves of the surgery. If there is disapproval, then less-than-optimal results may produce a reaction of, "See, I told you so!" that deepens the guilt and dissatisfaction of the patient.

Patients You Do Not Like (or Who Do Not Like You)

Regardless of the surgeon's personality, in life there are people you simply do not like or who do not like you. Accepting a patient you basically dislike is a serious mistake. A clash of personalities for whatever reason is bound to affect the outcome of the case, regardless of the actual quality of the postoperative result. No matter how interesting such a case may appear, it is far better to decline the patient.

The "Surgiholic"

A patient who has had various plastic surgery procedures performed and who is a "surgiholic" often is attempting to compensate for a poor self-image with repeated surgeries. In addition to the implications of such a personality pattern, the surgeon is also confronted with a more difficult anatomical situation because of the previous surgeries. He or she also risks unfavorable comparison with previous surgeons. Often, the percentage of achievable improvement is not worth the risk of the procedure.

Generally speaking, there is a clear risk–benefit ratio to every surgical procedure. If the risk–benefit ratio is favorable, the surgery should probably be encouraged and has a reasonable probability of success. If the risk–benefit ratio is unfavorable, then the reverse not only applies but the unintended consequences of the unfavorable outcome may turn out to be disproportionate to the surgical result. The only way to avoid this debacle is to learn how to distinguish those patients whose body image and personality characteristics make them unsuitable for the surgery that they seek.

THE WHEEL OF MISFORTUNE: EXPOSURES MOST LIKELY TO GENERATE CLAIMS

It should come as no surprise that the overwhelming majority of all malpractice claims lodged against plastic and reconstructive surgeons are concentrated in a handful of aesthetic surgery operations. Unlike other surgical specialists, the plastic surgeon attending a patient who seeks aesthetic improvement is not trying to make a sick patient well, but rather a well patient better. This not only places a heavier burden of responsibility on the operating surgeon but also subjects him or her to a broader range of possible reasons for unhappiness. Sources of dissatisfaction can range from a poor result to something as unpredictable as a patient's hidden emotional agenda or a simple communications failure.

Competitive pressures in the last few years have also blurred strict criteria for patient selection. As a result, it is not surprising to see a steadily upward trend in the frequency of claims against plastic and reconstructive surgeons. We have surveyed the genesis of patient complaints in a universe of plastic and reconstructive surgeons numbering roughly 700 across 15 years of experience. The loss experience in plastic surgery is notable for its frequency rather than its severity (the large number of claims alleging relatively minor damages). The average plastic surgeon reports a claim every 2.5 years. Although severity has not characterized plastic surgery's loss experience in the past, the trend is toward larger awards, particularly in those cases where an elective procedure has resulted in a fatal outcome. An important example is the claims arising out of large-volume suction-assisted lipectomy. This category of claims will be more carefully examined toward the conclusion of this chapter.

Scarring in General

Most surgeons assume the patient understands that healing entails formation of scar. Unfortunately, it is seldom discussed in the preoperative consultation. In plastic and reconstructive surgery, the appearance of the resulting scar can be the major genesis of dissatisfaction. It is imperative that the plastic surgeon obtains from the patient clear evidence of his or her comprehension that without scarring, there is no healing. The patient must be made to understand that healing qualities are as individual as the texture of one's hair or the color of one's eyes; it is built into genetic programming. Documentation of such conversation in the preoperative chart is most important.

Breast Reduction

The genesis of dissatisfaction most often involves the following:

• Unsatisfactory scar.
• Loss of a nipple or breast skin cover requiring revision.
• Asymmetry or "disfigurement."

Breast Augmentation

Litigation involving breast augmentation is even more common than breast reduction. Approximately 44% of all elective aesthetic surgery claims involve augmentation. Setting aside for the moment breast implants and autoimmune disease, the most frequent causes of dissatisfaction are as follow:

• Encapsulation with distortion and firmness.
• Wrong size (too little/too much).
• Infection.
• Repetitive surgeries and attendant costs.
• Nerve damage with sensory loss.

Facelift/Blepharoplasty

Facelift and blepharoplasty account for approx 11% of claims. The most common allegations are listed here:

• Excessive skin removal, resulting in a "stary" look.
• Dry eyes/inability to close.
• Nerve damage, resulting in distorted expression.
• Skin slough, resulting in excessive scarring and additional surgery.

The trend toward doing the vast majority of these patients on an outpatient basis deserves some comment. In a survey of blindness after blepharoplasty carried out by the author at The Doctors Company in 1999, it was discovered that the only trait all cases had in common was the fact that they were discharged very shortly after the termination of the outpatient surgery. Upon arrival at home, each did something to generate a sudden rise in blood pressure at the time of maximal reactive hyperemia as the epinephrine in the local anesthetic wore off (e.g., constipated bowel movement, sudden coughing fit, bending over and reaching down to tie shoes, etc.). It is imperative that all patients undergoing outpatient surgery involving undermining of heavily vascularized tissues be strictly warned not to undertake any maneuvers that will generate sudden elevations in blood pressure. Additionally, it is strongly recommended that no patient be discharged from an outpatient surgical facility until at least 3 hours have elapsed and there is evidence that all the local anesthetic effects have worn off.

Rhinoseptoplasty

Rhinoseptoplasty cases constitute approx 8% of the claims. Among the most common allegations are as listed here:

- Unsatisfactory result: improper performance allegations.
- Continued breathing difficulties.
- Asymmetry.

Unsatisfactory result is the most commonly seen by far. Of all the operations performed by plastic and reconstructive surgeons, this is regrettably the procedure with the highest degree of unpredictability. The problem is greatly aggravated by inappropriate patient-selection criteria. In these claims, there is almost universally a gap between the patient's expectations and the results obtained, even when the surgical outcome appears excellent. The inappropriate use of imaging devices or the showing of "brag books" containing only excellent results often causes patients to have unrealistic expectations. The clear implication is "this is the kind of work that I do, and this is what you can expect." Unfortunately, in many cases the actual result falls short of the promise, and the usual cycle is put into motion: surprise→disappointment→anger →perceived arrogance→increased avoidance→rising hostility→visit to the lawyer.

Abdominoplasty

Abdominoplasty with or without suction-assisted lipectomy represents approx 3% of claims. The most common allegations are:

- Skin loss with poor scars.
- Nerve damage.
- Inappropriate operation.
- Infection with postoperative mismanagement.

There is little question that the combination of suction-assisted lipoplasty prior to the actual abdominoplasty has significantly increased the morbidity of this operation and increased the number of claims in this category. There is a higher percentage of skin sloughs in those procedures when preceded by suction-assisted lipectomy.

Suction-Assisted Lipectomy

Suction-assisted lipectomy procedures, whether conventional or ultrasonic, have now become the single most requested elective aesthetic procedures in the United States. Approximately 145,000 of these procedures were performed in the year 1997, according to ASPRS statistics *(1)*. However, the rising popularity of this procedure has brought with it a host of problems. To begin with, because this is not a surgical procedure in the "traditional" sense, it is being performed by a wide variety of practitioners, some of them with no surgical background or clear understanding of the surgical anatomy involved. Second, it is a procedure most commonly done on an outpatient basis outside of the control of any regulatory authorities *(2)*. Additionally, with the advent of "tumescent" techniques, an unseemly race has developed to see who can suction out the most fat. The net result has been a dramatic rise in severe morbidity and fatal outcomes from high-volume liposuction. What is high volume? It is generally agreed that anything above 5000 cc of extracted fat constitutes high volume. The extraction of this amount of fat causes profound physiological changes, which in turn can lead to severe complications and/or fatal outcomes. The infusion of large amounts of fluid with even a weak concentration of lidocaine has also resulted in numerous fatal outcomes as a result of anesthetic overdose.

To make matters worse, these procedures are often combined with other prolonged operations. Our experience clearly indicates that when a patient has been under anesthesia for more than 6 hours undergoing multiple procedures, the percentage of complications and/or fatal outcome rises dramatically.

Overall, there are two categories of liability from conventional assisted lipectomy procedures:

1. Minor allegations:
   a. Disfigurement and contour irregularities
   b. Numbness
   c. Disappointment/dissatisfaction

2. Major allegations:
   a. Unrecognized abdominal perforation, resulting in disabling secondary surgery or death
   b. Lidocaine overdose with fatal outcome
   c. Pulmonary edema from over hydration
   d. Pulmonary embolism and death

The cavalier way in which this operation is sometimes performed requires rethinking, particularly when the amounts of fat extracted are major. In several venues in the United States, state medical regulatory authorities are beginning to take notice, and unless there is a significant downturn in the morbidity of this procedure, there will undoubtedly be some regulatory intervention to control the rising tide of misfortune.

Skin Resurfacing

Chemical peels and laser resurfacing constitute the next category of claims, constituting roughly 3%. The principle allegations here are as follows:

- Blistering/burns with significant scarring
- Infection/postoperative mismanagement
- Permanent discoloration postoperatively

Because of the unpredictability of individual healing characteristics, it is probably a good idea to do a "test patch" in an area that can be hidden (e.g., the back of the neck). Certainly, the documentation preceding this operation should contain clear warnings that quality of healing is linked to the individual's genetic makeup and cannot be predicted. The operator must make it clear to the patient that final color and texture determination is not in the hands of the surgeon and heavy make-up may be needed for an indeterminate period of time.

Miscellaneous

Approximately 5% of all complaints against plastic and reconstructive surgeons have to do with miscellaneous allegations, such as those listed here:

- Untoward reaction to medications or anesthesia
- Improper use of pre- or postoperative photos
- Sexual misconduct (doctor or employee)

There are certain common issues among all procedures performed by plastic and reconstructive surgeons that are commonly not brought to the attention of the patient in the preoperative consultations and often represent the triggering mechanism for a claim. They are as follows:

- Unexpected scarring
- Lack of adequate disclosure (tailored to the patient's level of understanding)
- General dissatisfaction (the patient's expectations were not met)

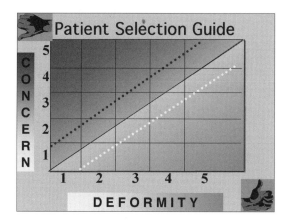

Fig.1. Criteria for patient selection.

PSYCHOLOGICAL AND PSYCHIATRIC
ASPECTS OF MODIFYING ANATOMY

The growing popularity of elective aesthetic surgery makes it imperative to establish clear criteria of patient selection. Who is the "ideal" candidate for aesthetic surgery? There is no such thing, but the surgeon should note any personality factors that will tend to enhance or detract from the physical improvements sought. The surgeon must differentiate between healthy and unhealthy reasons for seeking aesthetic improvement.

There are basically two categories that make the patient a poor candidate for elective aesthetic surgery. The first is anatomic unsuitability. The second is equally important, although more subtle—psychological inadequacy.

Strength of motivation is critical. It has a startlingly close relationship with the patient's satisfaction postoperatively. Furthermore, a strongly motivated patient will tend to have less pain, a better postoperative course, and a significantly higher index of satisfaction. Although these characteristics are impossible to predict with absolute accuracy, it is possible to establish some objective criteria for patient selection. These are illustrated in Fig. 1.

Figure 1 depicts a patient's objective deformity along the horizontal axis (as judged by the surgeon) vs the patient's degree of concern over that deformity (vertical axis; as perceived by the patient). Two opposite extremes emerge.

First, there is the patient with major deformity but minimal concern. This is a patient with an obvious major deformity in whom it is clear that any degree of improvement will be regarded with satisfaction.

Second, there is the patient with the minor deformity but extreme concern. In contrast, this is the patient with a deformity that the surgeon perceives to be minor but who demonstrates an inordinate degree of concern and emotional turmoil. These are the patients who are most likely to be dissatisfied with any outcome. The anxiety expressed over the deformity is merely a manifestation of inner turmoil, which is better served by a psychiatrist's couch than a surgeon's operating table.

Most who seek aesthetic surgery fit somewhere on a diagonal between the two contralateral corners shown in Fig. 1. The closer the patient comes to the upper left-hand corner, the more likely an unfavorably outcome is perceived, as is a visit to an attorney.

Effective Communication

Most litigation in plastic surgery has the common denominator of poor communication. This doctor–patient relationship can be shattered by the surgeon's arrogance, hostility, coldness (real or imagined), or simply by the fact that "he [or she] didn't care." There are only two ways to avoid such a debacle: (a) make sure that the patient has no reason to feel that way, and (b) avoid a patient who is going to feel that way no matter what is done.

Although the doctor's skill, reputation, and other intangible factors contribute to a patient's sense of confidence, rapport between patient and doctor is based on forthright and accurate communication. This will normally prevent the vicious cycle of disappointment, anger, and frustration by the patient and reactive hostility, defensiveness, and arrogance from the doctor, which deepens the patient's anger and ultimately may provoke a lawsuit.

Anger: A Root Cause of Malpractice Claims

Patients feel both anxious and bewildered when elective surgery does not go smoothly. The borderline between anxiety and anger is tenuous, and the conversion factor is uncertainty—fear of the unknown. A patient frightened by a postoperative complication or uncertain about the future may surmise: "If it is the doctor's fault, then the responsibility for correction falls on the doctor."

The patient's perceptions may clash with the physician's anxieties, insecurities, and wounded pride. The patient blames the physician, who in turn becomes defensive. At this delicate juncture, the physician's reaction can set in motion or prevent a chain reaction. The physician must put aside feelings of disappointment, anxiety, defensiveness, and hostility to understand that he or she is probably dealing with a frightened patient who is using anger to gain control.

The patient's perception that the physician understands that uncertainty and will join with him or her to help to overcome it may be the deciding factor in preserving the therapeutic relationship.

One of the worst errors in dealing with angry or dissatisfied patients is to try to avoid them. It is necessary to actively participate in the process rather than attempting to avoid the issue.

Body Dysmorphic Disorder

As the popularity of aesthetic surgery increases, one is reminded of the fairy tale that asks the question: "Mirror, mirror on the wall, who's the fairest of them all?" The number of patients finding comfort and solace in repetitive elective surgical procedures is growing. Beyond the unrealistic expectations of aesthetic correction, many patients are seeking surgery when the need for it is dubious at best. The physical change sought through surgery usually is more a manifestation of flawed body image than a measurable deviation from physical normality. Body dysmorphic disorder (BDD) represents a pathological preoccupation by the patient about a physical trait that may be within normal limits or so insignificant as to be hardly noticeable. However, to the patient it has become a consuming obsession.

As the trend to advertising and marketing cosmetic surgery grows worldwide there is greater probability that those living in the shadow of this diagnosis will eventually decide on the surgeon's scalpel as an answer to their problem rather than the psychiatrist's consultation.

Increasingly, we see traditional surgical judgment replaced either by financial consideration or plain ego on the part of the surgeon. Because patients with BDD never carry that diagnosis openly into the consultation with the plastic surgeon, medical disputes about the surgical outcome depend entirely on what was said vs what was understood.

In the best of all possible worlds, the prospective patient would project from the mind onto a screen exactly the changes he or she conceives for the surgeon to decide whether or not he or she can translate that image into reality. Lamentably, we are still many decades short of achieving such imaginary technology. It is easy for the well-meaning surgeon to be deceived about the patient's pathological motivation. It is also conceivable the physical deformity really is at the center of the patient's psychological fragility. There are many examples of beneficial change wrought through successful aesthetic corrective surgery. Nonetheless, statistically the odds for an unfavorable result and a claim are much greater when the disproportion between the objective deformity and the distress it creates in the patient is larger. The surgeon is cautioned to search for appropriate psychological balance and lean strongly against surgery in those where there is doubt.

At a time of convulsive change in the history of health care delivery in the United States, certain socioeconomic factors also come into play. With the rising number of practitioners in many specialties, competitive pressures have begun to affect patient selection criteria. There is a trend toward substitution economic considerations for surgical judgment. Because of recent constrictions on medical incomes, some practitioners see elective aesthetic surgery as the last area of practice unencumbered by either insurance or governmental restrictions. This has attracted individuals with inadequate qualifications. Even within the ranks of board certified plastic surgeons, the rising trend toward marketing and the need to sell surgery (which should always be motivated by the patient, not the surgeon) have further blurred patient selection criteria.

Although it is virtually impossible for a plastic and reconstructive surgeon to go through a 30- to 40-year career without a medical liability claim, it is possible to reduce the likelihood of this unpleasant experience by the application of simple principles: maintaining good communication and rapport with the patient through good times and bad, restricting your practice to those procedures on those with which you feel thoroughly comfortable, close and careful attention to documentation of your activities, and above all, the realization that a normal temperature and a valid credit card by themselves are very poor criteria for elective aesthetic surgery.

REFERENCES

1. ASPRS statistic, 1997.
2. TDC Guidelines for SAL, 2001/ASPS Standing Guidelines.

IV LEGAL REFORM AND HEALTH CARE

15 The Case for Legal Reform

Richard E. Anderson, MD, FACP

SUMMARY

The rising cost of claims has fueled a dramatic rise in the cost of medical malpractice insurance in the United States. Increasing severity has driven malpractice tort costs beyond $20 billion per year. A significant percentage of America's doctors are defendants in malpractice litigation and more than 600 new claims are initiated daily. Malpractice claims do not reliably identify "bad" doctors. In high-risk specialties, virtually all physicians are potential litigation targets. Other factors contributing to the increased cost of malpractice insurance include falling interest rates, higher costs for reinsurance, shrinking capacity, and judicial nullification of existing legal reforms.

More than a quarter century's experience with California's Medical Injury Compensation Reform Act (MICRA) statutes provides ample evidence that reforms are well defined and effective. In the absence of these reforms, it is predictable that the current crisis will worsen and access to fundamental medical services will be increasingly imperiled.

Key Words: Legal reform; tort reform; Medical Injury Compensation Reform Act (MICRA); premiums; frequency; severity; "bad" doctor; Harvard Medical Practice Study; Institute of Medicine; collateral source; periodic payments; caps; contingency fee; defensive medicine.

From: *Medical Malpractice: A Physician's Sourcebook*
Edited by: R. E. Anderson © Humana Press Inc., Totowa, NJ

INTRODUCTION

The past few years have seen significant increases in the cost of malpractice insurance in many parts of the United States *(1)*, making legal reform an issue of great significance to both doctors and health care consumers. Many physicians have been forced to curtail their practices, move to other venues, or even retire from the practice of medicine *(2–5)*. The issue has been extensively discussed and debated in the medical and legal press, the media in general, a number of state legislatures, and nationally by both Congress and the president. This chapter reviews the nature and extent of the problem, the relevant attributes of medical malpractice insurance, and the evidence that legal reforms can ameliorate the problem.

EXTENT OF THE PROBLEM

The expansion of tort law into new arenas of potential liability grew throughout the 20th century, particularly the latter half.

> *"... Tort law has existed here and abroad for centuries, of course. But until quite recently it was a backwater of the legal system, of little importance in the wider scheme of things. For all practical purposes, the omnipresent tort tax we pay today was conceived in the 1950s and set in place in the 1960s and 1970s by a new generation of lawyers and judges. In the space of twenty years they transformed the legal landscape, proclaiming sweeping new rights to sue. Some grew famous and more grew rich selling their services to enforce the rights that they themselves invented. But the revolution they made could never have taken place had it not had a component of idealism, as well. Tort law, it is widely and passionately believed, is a public-spirited undertaking designed for the protection of the ordinary consumer and worker, the hapless accident victim, the 'little guy.' Tort law as we know it is a peculiarly American institution. No other country in the world administers anything remotely like it"* (6).

Peter Huber, author of a seminal treatise on the expansion of liability law, refers to the attendant costs as the tort tax:

> *"It is one of the most ubiquitous taxes we pay, now levied on virtually everything we buy, sell and use. The tax accounts for 30 percent of the price of a stepladder and over 95 percent of the price of childhood vaccines. It is responsible for one-quarter of the price of a ride on a Long Island tour bus and one-third of the price of a small airplane. It will soon cost large municipalities as much as they spend on fire or sanitation services"* (6).

Responding to the same issues, Philip Howard has referred to "the death of common sense" *(7)*. He founded an organization named Common Good, which is dedicated to reforming America's legal system (http://cgood.org/). Common Good has this to say about the expansion of medical liability and the provision of health care in the United States:

> *"The lawsuit culture in modern America is creating a crisis in American healthcare. The broad perception that anyone can sue for almost anything has fundamentally altered the practice of medicine, eroding the quality and availability of healthcare."*

- Doctors are abandoning obstetrics and other specialties, and many are quitting practice altogether, because of legal exposure and costs;
- Honesty and candor, vital to improving health care systems and to delivering humane care, have been supplanted by a culture of legal fear;
- Vast resources are squandered in unnecessary 'defensive' medicine at the same time..." *(8)*.

Catherine Crier, lamenting the explosion in litigation wrote: "Trial work has become a major stand-alone business within the legal community. What was once the place for good advice about the worthiness of a claim has become a gristmill for expanding rights and remedies. To enterprising attorneys, there are few unmerited lawsuits. Traditionally, lawyers were officers of the court who zealously represented clients within legal and ethical boundaries. The interests of justice were paramount, such that intentionally misleading a jury or using discovery simply to wear down an opponent or drain his pocketbook was degrading to the practitioner and unethical as well. Using court pleadings or the media as a litigation tactic to destroy an opponent was unacceptable. Attorneys now regularly solicit clients, conjure up creative and nuisance filing, and delay the trial process, all to line their own pockets" *(9)*.

To get a sense of the magnitude of this phenomenon, it is interesting to note that if plaintiff attorneys were employed as members of a single corporation, it would have 50% more annual revenue than Microsoft and would be double the size of Coca-Cola *(10)*.

In general, the last decade of the 20th century was a period of rapid change and we, as a society, became accustomed to unprecedented numbers preceded by dollar signs. We live in a trillion-dollar economy. Mass tort litigation produces judgments of hundreds of billions of dollars and attorneys demand and receive billion-dollar fees. Twenty-two-year-olds who worked very hard for 18 months could find themselves Internet billionaires, and ballplayers could command hundred-million dollar contracts. Thus, the expansion of theories of liability has coincided with a significant monetary desensitization of the public mind. Jury verdicts in virtually all areas of the law have reached new heights with each succeeding year *(4,10)*.

Medical Context

It is not difficult to identify numerous factors affecting contemporary medical practice that have exacerbated medical malpractice liability within this broader cultural context. The foremost factor is managed care. Although ideally it offered the potential of cost savings, efficient medical practice patterns, and enhanced quality assessment and assurance, we have arrived at a place where virtually no major constituency is satisfied. Physicians and health care institutions are frustrated by reimbursement limitations, increased paperwork, and interruption of the traditional doctor–patient relationship. Patients decry access restrictions, reduced insurance coverage, and the need for frequent provider changes. Payors are unhappy with the resumption of significant increases in costs. Congress, seeing general dissatisfaction with the system, has attempted to pass legislation (i.e., 2001 Patients' Bill of Rights) that would have defined the public's rights under managed care and increased the potential for litigation directed against the managed care organizations themselves.

With virtually everyone disgruntled with significant aspects of their health care experience, the likelihood of malpractice suits increases. Because patient litigation against managed care organizations directly is limited by federal law (Employee Retirement Income Security Act [ERISA]), physicians often find they are targeted in litigation that might otherwise have been focused elsewhere. Suits alleging delayed diagnosis and failure to refer to appropriate specialists are especially potentiated because the real and imagined impediments of managed care in these areas resonate with juries.

Contemporary medical advances, especially in the realm of "medical miracles," are almost all technologically based. High-tech care is often low touch, and the skills needed to operate in this complex medical environment are not necessarily those that facilitate good bedside manner. Moreover, as the boundaries of possible medical intervention expand, expectations also rise. This produces potential litigation over adverse outcomes even in the most medically desperate circumstances.

Severity

Severity is an insurance term of art that refers to the cost of the average claim. By extension, it also connotes the range of potential adverse outcomes or the downside risk of taking a case to court. Since 1997, the increase in severity of medical malpractice litigation has been striking. The median malpractice verdict doubled from approx $500,000 to $1 million between 1997 and 2000 *(11)*, and the mean verdict increased from $1.97 million to $3.48 million over the same period *(12)*. The likelihood of a plaintiff's verdict exceeding $1 million increased from 34% in the period from 1994 to 1996 to 52% between 1999 and 2000 *(12)*. Therefore, it is not surprising that the total medical malpractice tort cost rose from $8.7 billion in 1990 to $20.9 billion in 2000—an increase of 140% *(13)*.

The amplification in the cost of the outlier verdict has been even greater. Texas recorded a judgment for $268 million. Several states have seen malpractice awards in excess of $100 million *(2)*. Until 2000, malpractice judgments were rarely, if ever, among the 10 largest in the United States in any given year. The Texas award made this list in 2000. In 2001, there were 2 medical malpractice claims among the top 10. Moreover, this list included a $312 million award against a nursing home for the care of a single patient, and a California jury returned a $3 billion verdict against the tobacco companies for the lung cancer death of a single smoker. Thus, 4 of the 10 largest judgments in the United States involved adverse health care outcomes for single individuals *(14)*. By 2002, fully half of the 10 largest awards in the United States involved health care outcomes of single individuals *(15)*.

Frequency

Frequency is another defined insurance term referring to the likelihood of a claim in a defined population of policyholders. For example, a frequency of 0.10 means that on the average, 10% of the group will report a claim every year or that each member will report a claim every 10 years. Frequency is very high among all physicians and averaged 15 to 16% in recent years, although the differences among specialties are significant (*see* Fig. 1). Approximately 55% of neurosurgeons report a claim (defined as a demand for payment) every year *(16)*. This means the average neurosurgeon would face a new claim every other year. For other high-risk specialties such as orthopedics, obstetrics, general surgery, and emergency medicine, frequency is around 30%. Even in "low-risk" specialties such as internal medicine,

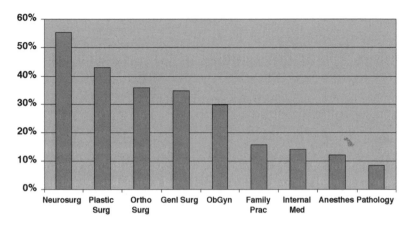

Fig. 1. Frequency by specialty from 1995 to 2001. (From The Doctors Company data on file.)

pathology, and anesthesiology, about 10% of policyholders will have a claim each year *(16)*.

Between 70 and 80% of all claims against physicians end without indemnity payment, meaning that the plaintiff receives nothing *(5)*. However, each claim requires a legal defense, and the attendant costs are high. In 2001, it cost a medical malpractice insurer an average of more than $23,000 in case-specific costs to close a nonmeritorious (zero pay) claim *(5)*. If such a claim had to go through a trial before a verdict for the defense, then the average cost was $85,718 *(5)*.

These costs are important drivers of premium rates. Although most malpractice claims end in vindication for the physician, the costs of the legal process are high. Allocated loss adjustment expense (ALAE) is the specific cost associated with an individual claim. The most important components are fees for defense attorneys and expert witnesses. ALAE does not include the overhead of the insurer in general or even the cost of running a claims department. It is important to note this cost driver. Ironically, all of these nonmeritorious claims have the paradoxical effect of driving down the cost of the average claim and increasing total claims expenses. The size of the average claim is best measured by specifying average paid claims. Without this seemingly obvious distinction, the large volume of nonmeritorious litigation can be distorted to appear to lower the cost of malpractice claims *(17)*.

THE ROLE OF MEDICAL
MALPRACTICE INSURANCE COMPANIES

Claims Losses

Although rising frequency and severity account for the dramatic increase in the annual cost of medical malpractice tort cases cited earlier *(13)*, there has been debate about whether this is adequate justification for the attendant increase in malpractice insurance premiums *(17,18)*. Because this issue has been central to legislative debate on the desirability of legal reform, it has been well studied from a number of viewpoints.

Conning & Co., a national insurance indemnity analyst, estimates that malpractice insurers will pay out approx $1.40 for every premium dollar collected in 2001 and 2002 *(19)*. Even with rate increases, Conning & Co. projects insurers will pay out $1.35 for each dollar collected in 2003 *(19)*. Similar figures have been presented by Tillinghast-Towers Perrin using data from A.M. Best *(20)*.

The preponderance of this loss comes from increased claims losses. Losses per doctor, the figure that would track individual physician premiums most closely, have risen considerably more than inflation, medical costs, or premiums themselves *(21)*. No relationship between premium costs and the general state of the economy was detectable *(21)*. To return to the medical malpractice insurance industry's 27-year average loss ratio (claims costs divided by premium), premiums would have required an increase of 59% in 2003 *(21)*. In every year since 1995, the cost of claims losses alone (without any accounting for expenses) has exceeded the total premium collected by malpractice insurers *(20)*.

In 2002, faced with a malpractice crisis in Florida, the governor appointed a blue ribbon commission to analyze the root causes of the problem and suggest solutions. The panel was chosen in a manner that assured impartiality and did not include physicians, attorneys, or insurers. It was composed of five university presidents who submitted a unanimous and unequivocal report.

> *"The primary cause of increased medical malpractice premiums has been the substantial increase in loss payments to claimants caused by increases in both the severity of judgments and the frequency of claims."*

> *"The Task Force finds that the lack of predictability in the market, combined with a trend toward increased damage judgments, has caused instability in the market which, in turn, has led to insurance*

carriers either increasing their premiums (often to a level above what independent doctors can afford) or withdrawing from the marketplace" (22).

The nonpartisan General Accounting Office (GAO), in its 2003 report to Congress on the cause of the rising cost of malpractice insurance, reached similar conclusions:

> *"Multiple factors have combined to increase medical malpractice premium rates over the past several years, but losses on medical malpractice claims appear to be the primary driver of increased premiums rates in the long term. Such losses are by far the largest component of insurer costs, and in the long run, premium rates are set at a level designed to cover anticipated costs"* (23).

The US Department of Health and Human Services issued a comprehensive report on the medical liability system and the quality of health care in the United States *(2)*. The department found: "Americans spend proportionately far more per person on the costs of litigation than any other country in the world. The excesses of the litigation system are an important contributor to 'defensive medicine'—the costly use of medical treatments by a doctor for the purpose of avoiding litigation. As multimillion-dollar jury awards have become commonplace in recent years, these problems have reached crisis proportions. Insurance premiums for malpractice are increasing at a rapid rate, particularly in states that have not taken steps to make their legal systems function more predictably and effectively" *(2)*. The report detailed rising claims losses as the main driver of increased premium rates and a threat to both quality and access in the health care system.

Accounting for Rate Increases: The Perfect Storm

Although claim costs comprise nearly 80% of an insurer's expenses *(23)*, there are additional factors that have contributed to the increase in malpractice premiums. Insurers must collect premium today to pay for the cost of claims in the future. In the case of malpractice claims, this gap may be long, because the average claim requires 3.5 years to resolve, and some claims are pending for as long as 10 years. It is the fiduciary responsibility of the insurance company to invest premium dollars prudently so that funds will be available to pay claims when needed. Approximately 80–90% of the average malpractice carrier's portfolio is invested in investment grade bonds, so investment income is heavily dependent on prevailing interest rates *(5,23)*. These have fallen considerably over the same period of time claims losses have been increasing. Therefore, there has been reduced income from investments to subsidize the cost of claims. Although virtually no malpractice insurer has suffered net negative investment returns, reduced investment income means that premium must cover a greater share of insurers' costs. The GAO has calculated that in the period from 2000 to 2002, premium rates would need to rise approx 7.2% to compensate for the fall in investment income *(23)*. However, this is a small percentage of overall rate increases, emphasizing the primary role played by rising claims losses.

In fact, the high returns of the 1990s enabled insurers to sell coverage for less than its actual cost by making up the difference with investment income. This worked well for the companies, which were able to grow despite intense price competition, and directly benefited policyholders, who received their insurance for less than cost. Unfortunately, when interest rates declined, the deficit created by the lost investment income added to premium increases necessitated by the rising cost of claims.

Faced with large losses, a number of malpractice insurers were forced into bankruptcy (notably PHICO, PIE, and Frontier, among others), and many more electively withdrew from the market, refusing to offer professional liability coverage at any price. St. Paul, a market leader in this field for more than two decades, was the largest and most important of these *(2)*. This shrank the capacity of the market as a whole to provide insurance for physicians and other health care providers.

Another factor adding to the upward pressure on malpractice premiums was a changed reinsurance market. Insurance companies buy reinsurance to prevent individual large losses from distorting results and to further spread the risk inherent in providing professional liability coverage in the first place. After September 11, the cost of this reinsurance rose significantly as reinsurers sought to recover from the estimated $75- to $100-billion cost of the tragic event. This meant that reinsurers demanded higher profit margins and more restricted coverages before they were willing to accept risk.

Finally, judicial nullification and threats to existing legal reforms contributed to the problem. State supreme courts in approximately a dozen states held the tort reforms approved by their respective state legislatures unconstitutional *(24)*. The loss of these reforms worsened the medical-legal environment for physicians and their insurers and is still another factor contributing to the rise in severity.

The Fallacy of the Bad Doctor

There would be less concern over the increase in malpractice premiums if the additional costs were born only by unqualified or negligent physicians. Indeed, one of the arguments for preserving the current system is that malpractice suits accurately identify these substandard doctors, thus performing an important societal function. However, the available data argue to the contrary. First, 70 to 80% of all malpractice claims today are found to be without merit (i.e., they close with no payment to the plaintiff) (5). So it cannot be reasonably argued that the existence of claims against a doctor is evidence of poor medical practice. This notion is underscored by the frequency data (Fig. 1) reviewed earlier, which indicate that 33 to 50% of all high-risk specialists face a claim every year. Expressed differently, the majority of malpractice claims in the United States today are filed against good doctors.

Further evidence that rising malpractice premiums are not caused by bad doctors can be found in a review of additional data. It is a reasonable rule of thumb in any given year that about 2% of physician-policyholders will account for approx 50% of the claims losses (16). This leads some to argue that eliminating these offenders would dramatically reduce premium rates. For this to be true, the same 2% of doctors would have to account for half the losses in succeeding years, and this is not the case. Although the rule of thumb is reliable enough, the doctors involved are different each year. Were this not true, other physicians would not practice with them, and insurance companies would certainly not insure them. This ratio is driven by the reverse causation: 2% of the plaintiffs receive 50% of all indemnity, and the 2% of doctors involved are not predictable, or in most cases even culpable (see below). This is not unexpected in a system so subject to the effects of outlier verdicts.

A review of the files of a national medical malpractice insurer indicates that less than 1% of its physician-policyholders have two paid claims over a 10-year period of time (16). The likelihood that a physician who has one paid claim will have a second in the succeeding decade is only one in five (16). Therefore, even paid claims do not reliably identify a group of physicians practicing substandard medicine.

Finally, the Harvard Medical Practice Study (25) looked at the actual litigation that arose from the more than 32,000 medical records they reviewed and concluded that there was no relationship whatever between the presence or absence of medical negligence and the outcome of malpractice litigation (26). The only variable correlated with the outcome of litigation was the degree of injury. Plaintiffs with the most serious injury were more likely to be successful in court, irrespective of whether the injury was caused by negligence.

Because the majority of malpractice claims are found to be without merit and the extent of injury is more strongly correlated with litigation outcome than with medical negligence, insurance companies cannot predict with any certainty the likelihood that an individual physician will incur malpractice liability in the future. This means premium rates must be predicated primarily on group, rather than individual, experience. In this context, medical specialty and geography (location of the practice) are more important determinants of rates than a physician's personal experience. Of course, there are exceptions (e.g., impaired physicians, extreme practice profiles, etc.), but exceptions are not the rule.

Using the extremes as an example, it is easy to see the limits of experience rating in the context of medical malpractice insurance. A physician with no claims could argue that his or her premium should be close to zero. On the other hand, following a single million-dollar claim, the physician's rate the following year could be many hundreds of thousands of dollars. Given the facts above, this would be illogical as well as unfair and would undermine the very notion of insurance. Therefore, in most cases the premium burden is evenly divided among physician groups with only modest experience-based discounts or surcharges actuarially creditable.

The Settlement Issue

Personal injury attorneys sometimes argue that outlier jury verdicts could be avoided if insurance companies settled claims more readily (27). There are several reasons that this is wrong. First, physician defendants win approx 80% of malpractice trials (5), making it difficult to argue that those claims should have been settled. Second, the physician, not the insurance company, is the defendant and usually retains the right to make any decision on settlement. In our legal system, the defendant is entitled both to the presumption of innocence and the right to a day in court. It is disingenuous for plaintiff attorneys to suggest that the courtroom has become too dangerous a venue for the exercise of one's legal rights. The alternative to a forced settlement should not be an unreasonable jury verdict. Finally, so-called "nuisance settlements" only encourage more litigation.

Insurance Companies and Markets

The plaintiff bar argues that the sharp rise in the cost of malpractice insurance is principally caused by exploitation of physicians and management incompetence by the companies that provide coverage. The facts do not support these allegations. Sixty percent of physicians are

insured in mutual companies owned by the policyholders themselves
(5). The remainder find coverage with commercial carriers, many of
which insure other risks unrelated to professional liability. The physician-owned companies are dedicated to providing malpractice coverage
for their policyholder-owners. These companies tend to be state-based,
although several have expanded regionally and a few nationally.

Several hundred companies write medical malpractice insurance in
the United States, but that figure may be misleading because only a
fraction of these are actively writing and the 20 largest medical liability
insurers accounted for 56% of malpractice premium in 2002 *(28)*. The
60% of physicians insured in physician-owned mutuals are spread
among approx 40 companies. When insurers perceive the medical-legal
environment as poor, they will be forced to reduce insurance writings or
leave the state entirely. A poor environment is basically defined as one
where premium rates fail to cover the risk of liability and a reasonable
return on investment. Forty-six companies, primarily commercial carriers but some mutuals as well, ceased writing this business between
2000 and 2002 *(28)*, typically for one of the following three reasons:

1. The company felt the business to be unprofitable, or more generally,
   that the practice of medicine had become uninsurable.
2. State regulators prohibited additional writing because of the precari-
   ous financial position of the company or regulatory violations.
3. Actual bankruptcy.

The exodus of such a large percentage of insurers from the market
has substantial costs for doctors, injured plaintiffs, and all health care
consumers. When a given market will not support enough insurers to
cover all doctors, the physicians will be unable to practice in that venue
and patients will be forced to travel long and potentially hazardous
distances to receive medical care. The insolvency of a malpractice
insurer is the worst possible outcome for both policyholders left uninsured and injured plaintiffs left uncompensated.

The following examples illustrated how this comes to pass. Between
1991 and 2000, malpractice insurers paid out $1.60 in losses and
expenses for each dollar of premium earned in Florida *(29)*. In 1999,
there were 66 active malpractice insurers in the state. By 2002, that
number had decreased to 12, and only 4 were accepting general new
business *(22)*. In Texas, where insurers paid out $1.35 for each dollar
of premium earned between 1991 and 2000 *(22)*, the number of active
insurers was reduced from 11 to 4 in 2002 *(30)*. No market can be
sustained very long by requiring its participants to lose money.

Table 1
Principal Provisions of MICRA

MICRA provisions	What they mean
$250,000 limit on noneconomic damages (i.e., pain and suffering).	No limit on actual damages. Limits only payment for pain and suffering.
Periodic payment of awards in excess of $50,000.	Damages are paid over the time period they are intended to cover, rather than as a lump sum.
Collateral source rule.	Prevents duplicate collection of damages already paid by a third party.
Contingency fee limitation.	Controls the size of contingency fees using a sliding scale. For a $1 million award, an attorney is limited to $221,000, plus expenses.

The value of legal reforms in stabilizing insurance markets will be discussed in the next section.

THE VALUE OF LEGAL REFORMS

Although legal reform has been endlessly and repetitively debated in professional, legislative, and media forums across the United States in recent years, in truth we have more than a quarter century of experience and data, and relatively clear answers are available *(2,5,22,27, 31–34)*.

The first malpractice crisis crystallized in California in 1975. Between 1968 and 1974, the number of malpractice claims doubled and the number of losses in excess of $300,000 increased 11-fold *(35)*. Insurers were paying out $180 for each $100 of premium they collected *(35)*. Most commercial insurers concluded that the practice of medicine was uninsurable, and they refused to provide malpractice coverage at any price. Faced with the prospect of either no malpractice insurance at all or premiums that were not affordable, physicians selectively withheld medical services, and access to care was threatened throughout the state. Doctors marched on the state capital. A special session of the California legislature was called to deal with the crisis. The result was the Medical Injury Compensation Reform Act of 1975 (MICRA; *see* Table 1).

The most important of the MICRA reforms is a $250,000 cap on noneconomic damages. California does not limit awards for economic damages, but capping pain and suffering awards takes the lottery aspect out of malpractice litigation. Economic damages are defined broadly and include lost wages, medical and nursing care, and rehabilitation.

The second major MICRA reform is the provision for periodic payments. This allows damage awards to be paid over the period of time that they are intended to cover. Such a rule means injured patients will actually receive payment in the timeframe in which it is needed. Moreover, the time value of money allows the insurance system to accommodate even very large judgments without facing insolvency.

The third major MICRA reform is the collateral source rule. This prevents duplicate collection for the same damages. For example, if an injured patient has already had lost wages or medical costs covered by disability or medical insurance, recovery may not be duplicated in a malpractice award. This is not only equitable but also avoids using the tort system, with its 72% transaction tax (2), as a mechanism for funding basic services that have already been covered.

Fourth, there are modest limits on attorneys' contingency fees. MICRA provides for a sliding scale: a plaintiff attorney keeps 40% of the first $50,000 of an award but "only" 21% (plus expenses) of a $1 million judgment. This rules protects patients, allowing more of an award to actually reach the injured patient. The difference is significant. A patient with a $1 million award in a state with a contingency fee of 40% must give $400,000 (plus expenses) to his or her attorney as compared to $221,000 (plus expenses) under MICRA.

These reforms have reduced California malpractice premiums by 40% in constant dollars since 1975, or less than 3% per year uncorrected for inflation (16). On average, California's malpractice premiums have risen at a rate of only one-third the national average (Fig. 2 [29]).

There are considerable data that a $250,000 cap on noneconomic damages reduces malpractice premiums by 25 to 30% (2,28,36), and experience in California, Colorado, and other states is confirmatory.

The mirror image of the positive effect of real reform can be seen in the experience of states that had caps on noneconomic damages that were invalidated by their state supreme courts. Ohio enacted MICRA-like reforms in 1975, but the Ohio Supreme Court nullified these in 1985. Malpractice insurance rates fell steadily until 1982, when the law was challenged in the courts. Since 1985, Ohio malpractice premiums have once again increased significantly and the state is dealing with a

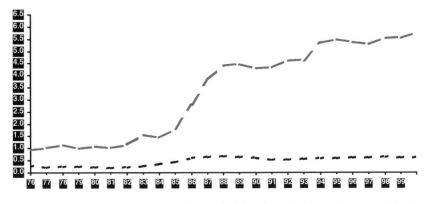

Fig. 2. Savings from MICRA reforms: California vs US premiums for 1976–2000. (From ref. *5*.)

new malpractice crisis *(33,37)*. In 2003, Ohio approved a new set of reforms in an effort to ameliorate the growing problem.

The experience in Oregon is even more dramatic. The state legislature capped noneconomic damages at $500,000 in 1987. The Oregon Supreme Court nullified this law in 1998. By 2000, malpractice indemnities in the state had increased 400% compared to 1998 *(38)*.

Alabama, Georgia, Illinois, Kansas, New Hampshire, North Dakota, and Washington have also had tort reforms nullified by their state supreme courts *(4)*. Today, Georgia, Illinois, Oregon, and Washington are among the 19 states facing a professional liability crisis *(4)*.

Other states have passed reforms that did not include damage caps. New York did so in 1975, 1981, and 1986 with no observable improvement in the malpractice insurance situation *(33)*. Florida and Texas have repeated similar experiences *(24)*, and in 2003 both state legislatures attempted to remedy the deteriorating medical-legal climate in their state with new reforms that do include caps on noneconomic damages.

A work group of the American Academy of Actuaries concluded that to be effective, a package of medical malpractice reforms must include a $250,000 per injury limit on noneconomic damages and a collateral source offset *(33)*. They found that reforms worked best when implemented together as a comprehensive program. Most significantly, they confirmed that porous caps with built-in exceptions or multipliers and peripheral reforms that do not include the fundamental elements of MICRA are predictably ineffective.

Beyond this, there is considerable additional evidence bearing on the effectiveness of legal reform in reducing malpractice premium rates. States with $250,000 or $350,000 limits on noneconomic damages had average premium increases only one-third as large as those in states without caps between 2000 and 2001 *(2,39)*. California's experience over the preceding quarter century stands as firm testimony to these data.

In 2002, the nonpartisan Congressional Budget Office estimated that the MICRA-based reforms contained in House Resolution 4600 (which failed to pass the Senate) would have lowered malpractice insurance premiums by 25 to 30% *(40)*.

Milliman USA analyzed medical malpractice claims in the 15 largest states from 1990 to 2001 and concluded that caps on noneconomic damages reduced medical malpractice loss costs for physicians *(41)*. In this study, reform states like California and Colorado saw loss costs reduced 48 and 31%, respectively. In contrast, New York's loss cost per physician stood at 300% compared to California, and Pennsylvania's stood at 328%. In an earlier study, Milliman had estimated that a $250,000 cap on noneconomic damages in New York would reduce premium levels by 29% *(32)*.

Perhaps the most comprehensive study of this issue ever undertaken was that delivered by the Governor's Select Task Force on Healthcare Professional Liability Insurance in Florida in 2002 *(22)*. Testimony ran to 13 volumes and included physicians, lawyers, insurance industry representatives, regulators, legal scholars, professional organizations, and concerned citizens. The final report exceeds 300 pages and contains more than 1300 citations. However, its conclusions were clear and unanimous. The report takes note of Florida's past history of unsuccessful reform and concludes that:

> *"A cap on non-economic damages of $250,000 per incident limited only to healthcare professional liability cases is the only available remedy that can produce a necessary level of predictability ... without the inclusion of a cap on potential awards of non-economic damages in the package, no legislative reform plan can be successful in achieving a goal of making medical malpractice insurance affordable and available, and thereby controlling increases in healthcare costs and promoting improved access to healthcare"* (22).

The authors noted that Florida's unsuccessful previous attempts at reforms that did not include such a cap "are nothing more than a failed litany of alternatives" *(22)*.

The National Association of Insurance Commissioners (NAIC) studied the market for medical malpractice insurance to evaluate the current crisis in 2003 *(28)*. Its conclusions, made independently and with access to the considerable state statutory data and experience, are in accord with those detailed previously. It found rising premium rates to be primarily a function of increasing claims costs. In addition, they found these problems were impeding public access to essential health care. They made six recommendations for states to consider when addressing these issues, including a $250,000 cap on noneconomic damages, a periodic payments provision, and collateral source reform. In addition, they recommended consideration of reforms to limit nonmeritorious claims, "bad faith" claims (*ex post facto* litigation alleging failure to make a timely settlement), and exploration of mechanisms that would add more predictability to insurers' loss costs *(28)*.

There is ample evidence that the MICRA reforms have had a substantial impact on the availability and cost of malpractice insurance. In assessing the cost of the current crisis, we should also review the impact of defensive medicine and reduced access to care.

Defensive Medicine

In addition to its obvious direct impact, the tidal wave of malpractice litigation extracts a severe indirect toll on practicing physicians *(42,43)*, forcing many doctors to regard patients as potential adversaries and leading to the practice of defensive medicine. By definition, defensive medicine is unnecessary and consists of interventions that do not benefit the patient but are meant to protect the physician from litigation. Therefore, defensive medicine is always wasteful. The facile argument that perhaps a degree of defensive medicine would be salutary for our health care system is thus clearly invalid. Unfortunately, one can argue that virtually all medicine in the United States is to some degree defensive *(43)*. Medical standards of care have been replaced by medical-legal standards, physician judgment has been devalued, and the value of medical chart documentation set above the actual benefit to the patient. The standard of care in the community is not necessarily the most rational or the one with best supporting evidence but rather the one that keeps physicians out of court. Two examples of this phenomenon nationally are the high rate of Cesarean sections (C-sections) and high percentage of mammograms interpreted as suspicious for breast cancer *(43)*. The United States has a much higher C-section rate than any other developed country, with no improvement in birth outcomes. This phenomenon is clearly caused by litigation pressure. Similarly, the rate of false-positive mammograms in the United States is twice that in other developed countries, again without improving the cancer detection rate. In another example of litigation-biased decision making, cardiac surgeons have been accused of gaming risk selection of patients to improve outcome data, limiting surgical access for the highest risk patients *(44)*.

Even ignoring the emotional burden and the damage caused by litigation-scared physicians practicing angry or hurt, the dollar costs are enormous. In 1996, Kessler and McClellan *(45)* estimated the cost of defensive medicine at $50 billion and argued that extending current malpractice reforms to all the states would reduce health care costs by 5 to 9%. More recently, the Department of Health and Human Services calculated the savings at $60 to $108 billion per year *(2)*. Although these may be the best estimates available, they are extremely conservative. These numbers reflect the reduced cost of health care in states with effective tort reform compared to states lacking such reforms. California, inherently a litigious state, has a frequency of malpractice litigation that is about 50% above the national average *(16)*, despite MICRA. Although the data indicate that effective tort reforms reduce the practice of defensive medicine, it is clearly not eliminated. This would suggest that the true costs are considerably higher than indicated by this methodology.

Because financing the cost of health care in the United States today is a zero-sum game, these direct and indirect costs of the malpractice crisis must be subtracted from funds available to fund the care of the uninsured and underinsured *(2,5,31)*, and for medical research and innovation. Reasonable limits on noneconomic damages, by reducing both the direct costs of malpractice insurance and the cost of defensive medicine, would save enough money to fund a prescription drug benefit for Medicare beneficiaries and facilitate insurance coverage for millions of uninsured Americans *(2)*.

Access to Care

As direct and indirect cost drivers increase the price of health care, it becomes unaffordable for an incremental number of patients. As the cost of malpractice insurance increases, it becomes unaffordable for an incremental number of doctors, other health care providers, and medical institutions, effectively preventing them from delivering medical services. As the fear of malpractice litigation and the consequent increase in malpractice insurance rates affect physician behavior, doctors become incrementally more averse to high-risk procedures, difficult patients, and more litigious venues. They also become incrementally more susceptible to practices with more benefit in litigation avoidance than patient care. The same pressures will incrementally affect the choice of specialties by medical students and investment in medical facilities and medical research *(46)*.

None of this would appear to be particularly controversial; however, for several reasons it is difficult to be precise about the magnitude of these effects or to define the exact tipping point for individual physicians, specialties, facilities, or communities. First, "affordability" is a relative concept. Second, there are many contributors to the price of health care. Third, there are no adequately defined and scaled metrics for analysis as costs and their consequential pressures continue to rise. Moreover, there is an important personal factor in evaluating the access to care issue that goes beyond statistical analysis. If it is your obstetrician who is unavailable, then you have an access to care crisis. If the trauma center closest to the scene of your accident is closed, then you have an access to care problem. If there is no neurosurgeon available in your community following your head injury, then you have an access to care issue.

The Florida Select Task Force looked carefully at access to care because they felt it to be the most important reason for reform of laws governing medical malpractice litigation. The Task Force Report provides 33 pages (pp. 69–102 in ref. *22)* of examples where the cost of malpractice insurance threatens or has already reduced access to care. Again, their conclusion was unequivocal:

> *"The concern over litigation and the cost and lack of medical malpractice insurance have caused doctors to discontinue high-risk procedures, turn away high-risk patients, close practices, and move out of the state. In some communities, doctors have ceased or discontinued delivering babies and discontinued hospital care"* (22).

On the other hand, with effective tort reform:

> *"Physicians and hospitals will not be compelled to reduce or eliminate services, particularly those involving high risk. High-cost and low-income groups in particular will benefit. Lower malpractice insurance rates increase the willingness of physicians and hospitals to provide treatments that carry a relatively high risk of failure but offer the only real prospect of success for seriously ill patients"* (22).

Three separate arms of the federal government reached similar conclusions. The Agency for Healthcare Research and Quality found that states with caps on noneconomic damages had 12% more physicians per capita than states without these reforms *(47)*.

The US Department of Health and Human Services found:

> *"This is a threat to health care quality for all Americans. Increasingly, Americans are at risk of not being able to find a doctor when they most need one because the doctor has given up practice, limited the practice to patients without health conditions that would increase the litigation risk, or moved to a state with a fairer legal system where insurance can be obtained at a lower price"* (2).

The GAO compared health care access in five states with rapidly rising medical malpractice premiums to four states with more stable medical-legal environments *(3)*. The GAO found:

> *"Actions taken by health care providers in response to rising malpractice premiums have contributed to localized health care access problems in the five states reviewed with reported problems. GAO confirmed instances in the five states of reduced access to hospital-based services affecting emergency surgery and newborn deliveries in scattered, often rural areas where providers identified other long-standing factors that also affect the availability of services. Instances were not identified in the four states without reported problems"* (3).

There are many specific examples of compromised health care caused by our litigation system. This list is not meant to be comprehensive but rather to show both the widespread nature of the problem as well as its immediacy.

- Access to Pap smears for the detection of cervical cancer is threatened because lawsuits demand an impossible to achieve zero error rate *(48)*.
- More than 12% of obstetricians/gynecologists across the country have ceased delivering babies, and nearly twice that number have reduced their exposure to high-risk obstetric care *(48)*.
- Abbott Laboratories withdrew its participation in a National Institutes of Health clinical trial designed to test a vaccine to prevent HIV-positive mothers from infecting their unborn children because of fear of liability *(48)*.
- Dupont restricted the sale of raw materials to manufacturers of artificial blood vessels, heart valves, and sutures to avoid litigation over the use of these devices *(48)*.
- The northern panhandle of West Virginia lost all neurosurgical services for about 2 years when the neurosurgeons who served the area

either left or stopped providing services because of malpractice pressures *(3)*.

- Pregnant women in parts of Mississippi had to travel 65 miles to deliver after the local hospital was forced to closed its obstetrical unit *(3)*.
- The only Level I trauma center in Nevada was forced to close for nearly 2 weeks when 60 orthopedic surgeons refused to provide services to protest the cost of malpractice insurance *(3)*.
- Parts of Pennsylvania have suffered a significant physician exodus because of high malpractice insurance costs; 44 occurred in Delaware County in 1 year alone *(2)*.
- In Ohio, a urologist would have had to spend 7 months of his yearly income simply to cover the cost of malpractice insurance *(2)*.
- Sixty-five percent of New Jersey hospitals report that physicians are leaving because of the cost of malpractice insurance *(2)*.
- Community clinics report increasing difficulty finding volunteer physicians because of liability fears *(2)*.

Finally, it is instructive to review California's quarter century experience with MICRA to measure its effect on health care access. William Hamm, the former legislative analyst for the California Assembly, analyzed the effect of MICRA on health care costs for safety net providers and Medi-Cal *(49)* (California's version of Medicaid for low-income Californians). He found that MICRA:

- Provided significant cost savings to teaching and safety net hospitals.
- Saved as much as $826 million for Medi-Cal.
- Reduced the practice of defensive medicine, which otherwise increases medical costs.
- Produced significant savings for nonprofit and community clinics, which otherwise would find it necessary to reduce services or increase fees.

Looking at California's health care system more generally *(31)*, he found the following:

- MICRA played a critical role in promoting access to health care for high-cost and low-income groups.
- MICRA's favorable impact on losses and malpractice insurance premiums reduced the cost of health care in California.
- Cost-savings are reflected in health insurance premiums, making health insurance benefit programs more affordable to businesses, particularly small businesses.
- Reduced "malpractice pressure" will increase the supply of physicians in California.

- Lower malpractice insurance premiums contribute to the viability of community hospitals.
- Lower malpractice insurance rates increase the willingness of physicians and hospitals to provide treatments that carry a relatively high risk of failure but offer the only real prospect of success for seriously ill patients.
- MICRA has improved California's access to health care by reducing provider fees, discouraging treatment that inflates costs but does not improve outcomes, and dampening malpractice pressure that tends to reduce the supply of physicians—particularly in key specialty areas, such as obstetrics, and underserved communities, such as rural areas and inner cities.

What can we conclude about rising malpractice premiums and access to care? Eighty-four percent of Americans believe availability and quality of health care is threatened by rising malpractice premiums *(50)*. This is a strikingly high figure for any poll. It is also a particularly sharp counterpoint to the notion that malpractice suits are effective in identifying substandard medical care (*see* The Fallacy of the Bad Doctor section on p. 209).

Until the entire health care system breaks down completely under the pressure of malpractice litigation, the threat to health care access will be incremental, felt differently by individual doctors, patients, and communities. However, it is clearly a significant problem. This is especially true if it is your family's health that is compromised.

SUMMARY AND CONCLUSIONS

The crisis in medical malpractice insurance has arisen in a context of a dramatic increase in the overall scope and cost of litigation in the United States. However, there are a number of factors specific to medicine that have accelerated this event. They have in common an undermining of the doctor–patient relationship and include dissatisfaction with managed care, the increased use of technology in medicine, weakening the personal bonds between physician and patient, and rising expectations for medical interventions.

Increasing severity has led to an unprecedented increase in the cost of malpractice claims, now surpassing $20 billion per year and still rising rapidly. A high percentage of America's physicians are currently in litigation and 600 new claims are opened daily. In the highest risk specialties, 33 to 50% of all practitioners report a claim every year. Even worse, there is no evidence that malpractice suits reliably identify "bad" doctors. Indeed, we have considerable data to the contrary. Litigation outcomes are correlated with patient injury rather than medical negligence, and even paid claims are only weakly predictive of future litigation problems for individual physicians. Certain specialties have become repetitive targets for malpractice suits because of the serious nature of the clinical problems rather than the quality of the medicine being practiced.

Although several factors have contributed to the increased cost of malpractice insurance, the rising cost of claims is by far the most important. Falling interest rates, higher costs for reinsurance, shrinking capacity, and judicial nullification of existing legal reforms are also issues.

Since 1975, we have had direct experience with various legal reforms and clear knowledge of which of these are effective and which are not. It is best to effectuate legal reform as part of a comprehensive package based on California's MICRA experience. A $250,000 cap on noneconomic damages is most important, but collateral source reform, a periodic payments rule, and control of attorney contingency fees are also important. Other reforms may be appropriate and useful, but a quarter century of experience indicates they will have much less impact than the MICRA statutes.

In the absence of these reforms, it is predictable that the cost of malpractice insurance will continue to rise, as will the cost of medical care in general, defensive medicine will increase, and access to fundamental health care will be increasingly imperiled.

REFERENCES

1. Medical Liability Monitor. 2003 rate survey shows rates still on the rise, underwriting tougher, no end in sight. Medical Liability Monitor. Vol. 28, 2003:1–20.
2. US Department of Health and Human Services. Confronting the New Health Care Crisis: Improving Health Care Quality and Lowering Costs by Fixing Our Medical Liability System. Washington, DC, 2002:1–28.
3. United States General Accounting Office. Medical Malpractice: Implications of Rising Premiums on Access to Health Care. Washington, DC, 2003:57.
4. AMA. Medical Liability Reform—NOW! Chicago, 2003:29.
5. Harming Patient Access to Care: Implications of Excessive Litigation. Subcommittee on Health, Committee on Energy and Commerce, US House of Representatives. Washington, DC: US Government Printing Office, 2002:160.
6. Huber PW. Liability: The Legal Revolution and Its Consequences. New York, NY: Basic Books, 1988.
7. Howard PK. The Death of Common Sense. New York, NY: Warner Books, 1994.
8. Common Good. Common Good Petition. Website: http://cgood.org. Accessed: 12/5/03.
9. Crier C. The Case Against Lawyers. Broadway Books, 2003.

224   Anderson

10. Center for Legal Policy. Trial Lawyers Inc. Manhattan Institute, 2003:31.
11. Bagin G. Medical Malpractice Verdict and Settlement Study Released. Horsham, PA: Jury Verdict Research, 2002.
12. Jury Verdict Research. 2001 Current Award Trends in Personal Injury, 2002.
13. Tillinghast-Towers Perrin. US Tort Costs: 2002 Update, 2003.
14. Model's jury award top verdict. Lawyers Weekly USA 2001.
15. Record Tobacco Verdict Tops Year's Large Awards. Lawyers Weekly USA, 2002.
16. The Doctors Company data on file. Napa, CA 2002.
17. Hunter JR, Doroshow J. Premium Deceit–The Failure of "Tort Reform" to Cut Insurance Prices. New York: Center for Justice & Democracy, 2002.
18. Nace BJ, Stewart LS. Straight Talk on Medical Malpractice: American Trial Lawyers Association, 1994:20.
19. Conning Research & Consulting I. Medical Malpractice: Anatomy of a Crisis 2003, 2003.
20. Hurley JD. A new crisis for the Med Mal market? Emphasis (Tillinghast), 2002: 4;2–5.
21. Ramachandran R. Did Investments Affect Medical Malpractice Premiums?: Brown Brothers Harriman Insurance Asset Management Group, 2003.
22. Governor's Select Task Force. Governor's Select Task Force on Healthcare Professional Liability Insurance. Orlando, FL: University of Central Florida, 2003.
23. United States General Accounting Office. Medical Malpractice Insurance: Multiple Factors Have Contributed to Increased Premium Rates. Washington, DC, 2003:67.
24. American Tort Reform Association. ATRA's Tort Reform Record, 2003.
25. Weiler PC, Hiatt HH, Newhouse JP, Johnson WG, Brennan TA, Leape LL. A Measure of Malpractice. Cambridge, MA: Harvard University Press, 1993.
26. Brennan TA, Sox CM, Burstin HR. Relation between negligent adverse events in the outcomes of medical malpractice litigation. N Engl J Med 1996:335; 1963–1967.
27. Anderson R. Defending the Practice of Medicine. Arch Intern Med 2003, 164.
28. National Association of Insurance Commissioners. Medical Malpractice Insurance: A Study of Market Conditions, 2003, pp. 28, 34.
29. NAIC. National Association of Insurance Commissioners 1999 Profitability Study, 1999.
30. Texas Department of Insurance. Medical Malpractice Insurance: Overview and Discussion, 2002.
31. Hamm WG. An Analysis of Harvey Rosenfield's Report: "California's MICRA": LECG, 1997, p. 1–25.
32. Biondi RS, Quintilian K. Medical Liability Mutual Insurance Company Projected Effect on New York Professional Liability Costs of Capping Noneconomic Damages: Milliman & Robertson, 1995.
33. American Academy of Actuaries. Medical Malpractice Reform in California, Ohio and New York. Contingencies, 1995, pp. 22–25.
34. US Congress Office of Technology Assessment. Impact of legal reforms on medical malpractice costs. Washington, DC: US Government Printing Office, 1995:64.
35. Keene B. California's medical malpractice crisis: Health Care Liability Alliance, 2003, pp. 1–13.

36. American Academy of Actuaries. Medical Malpractice Tort Reform: Lessons from the States, 1996.

37. Excerpts of Reports Received by the American Tort Reform Association on the Crisis in Medical Liability: American Medical Association, 2002.

38. Oregon Med Mal 1996–2001 ($000s). Sheshunoff Info Services: NW Physicians Mutual Insurance Company, 2002.

39. Medical Liability Monitor. Trends in 2002 Rates for Physicians' Medical Professional Liability Insurance. Chicago, 2002:1–16.

40. Congressional Budget Office. Cost Estimate for HEALTH Act of 2002, 2002, pp. 1–10.

41. Milliman USA. Milliman USA Analysis Sees Savings for Professional Medical Malpractice Costs. New York, NY, 2003.

42. Charles SC, Wilbert JR, Franke KJ. Sued and non-sued physicians' self-reported reactions to malpractice litigation. Am J Psychiatry 1985:142;437–440.

43. Anderson R. Billions for defense: the pervasive nature of defensive medicine. Arch Intern Med 1999;159:2399–2402.

44. Schneider E, Epstein A. Influence of cardiac-surgery performance reports on referral practices and access to care. A survey of cardiovascular specialists. N Engl J Med 1997;335:251–256.

45. Kessler DP, McClellan M. Do doctors practice defensive medicine? QJ Econ 1996:111;353–390.

46. American Medical Association. Medical students not immune to nation's medical liability crisis. AMA Website 2003.

47. Hellinger F, Encinosa W. The Impact of State Laws Limiting Malpractice Awards on the Geographic Distribution of Physicians: Agency for Healthcare Research and Quality, US Department of Health and Human Services, 2003.

48. Health Coalition on Liability and Access. The Health Care Liability System Bars Access to Health Care, 2003.

49. Hamm WG. How the MICRA Cap Influences Health Care Costs for Safety Net Providers and Medi-Cal: LECG, 1999;1–13.

50. Health Coalition on Liability and Access. Americans Believe Access to Health Care Threatened by Medical Liability Crisis. Washington, DC, 2003.

16 Health Policy Review

Medical Malpractice

David M. Studdert, LLB, ScD, MPH,
Michelle M. Mello, JD, PhD, MPhil,
and Troyen A. Brennan, MD, JD, MPH

SUMMARY

Since the 1980s, empirical analyses of the system of medical malpractice have revealed that it largely fails to provide reasonable compensation for injured individuals, or to provide appropriate incentive for safety and prevention. The most promising approaches for reform involve fundamental system changes rather than tinkering with tort doctrine.

Key Words: Standard of care; Harvard Medical Practice Study; patient safety; tort reform; system reform.

INTRODUCTION

Few issues in health care spark ire and angst like medical malpractice litigation. Physicians revile malpractice claims as random events that visit unwarranted expense and emotional pain on competent, hardworking practitioners. Commentators lament the "lawsuit lottery" that provides windfalls for some patients but no compensation for

From: *Medical Malpractice: A Physician's Sourcebook*
Edited by: R. E. Anderson © Humana Press Inc., Totowa, NJ

the vast majority of patients injured by medical care *(1,2)*. Within the health care industry, there is a near-universal belief that malpractice litigation has long since surpassed sensible levels and major tort reform is overdue.

Yet the litigation presses forward. Plaintiff attorneys and some consumer groups interpret providers' grievances as little more than predictable chafing from a profession unaccustomed to external policing. They view litigation as an indispensable form of protection against medical carelessness. Trial attorneys' responses to recent research on medical errors illustrates their self-image as champions of patient safety: new knowledge of the burden of medical error is seen as vindication of the battles fought on behalf of patients, and the imperative such findings announce is clear—more litigation *(3)*.

With a malpractice crisis now spreading across the United States, it is timely to review the current situation in light of the liability system's goals, previous crises, and available evidence on system performance. A survey of the field yields a picture of a system that has internal logic but falls far short of its social goals of promoting safer medicine and compensating wrongfully injured patients.

SYSTEM FRAMEWORK AND GOALS

Malpractice law is part of tort law, or personal injury law. To prevail in tort lawsuits, the plaintiff must prove that the defendant owed a duty of care to the plaintiff, the defendant breached that duty by failing to adhere to the standard of care expected, and this behavior caused an injury to the plaintiff *(4)*.

The standard traditionally used to evaluate whether the breach in question rises to the level of negligence is medical custom—what would be expected of a reasonable practitioner in similar circumstances. Custom is determined primarily through the testimony of experts in the same field as the defendant, although some encapsulations of expert opinion, such as practice guidelines, may also be used *(5,6)*. In at least 20 states, there has been a discernible shift in recent years away from custom and toward more independent determinations by the court of whether the defendant deviated from "reasonable" conduct *(7)*.

The social goals of malpractice litigation are threefold: to deter unsafe practices, compensate persons injured by negligence, and exact corrective justice *(4)*. Theoretically, lawsuits deter physicians by reminding those who wish to avoid the emotional and financial costs of litigation that they must take care *(8)*. With respect to compensation, tort theory posits that there are strong fairness and efficiency reasons for forcing the party at fault for an injury to bear the associated costs, including lost earnings, medical bills, and pain and suffering.

Clinicians and health care facilities are well-placed to bear injury costs because they are able to pool risk and resources through insurance *(9)*. Nearly all hospitals and physicians carry coverage that is fairly broad, often through lines of insurance separated into doctors on the one hand and institutions and their employees on the other. The cost of insurance coverage for hospitals is typically linked to claims history from year to year ("experience rating"). On the other hand, physicians, generally are not "risk rated" unless they have been chronically sued, in which case they may be forced into high-cost insurers or have trouble obtaining any coverage *(10)*. Experience rating of physicians is very difficult given the randomness of claims and the very limited predictive value of one or two claims in high-risk specialties. In recent years, anecdotal evidence suggests that some insurers in tort crisis states are declining to renew policies for physicians with even a single claim.

Several patient and physician characteristics have been linked to patients' decisions to bring malpractice claims, most notably patient dissatisfaction *(11,12)* and physician communication and interpersonal skills *(13,14)*. However, once the patient has decided to sue, the plaintiff attorney becomes the pivotal player in determining the volume and type of malpractice lawsuits. The plaintiffs' attorney acts as the system's turnstile because claims rarely move forward without the stewardship of counsel. Most plaintiffs' attorneys work on a contingency fee basis, taking a percentage of the award as a fee (usually around 35%) and taking nothing if the defendant prevails. Because they must absorb the costs of managing litigation regardless of the outcome, plaintiff attorneys have an incentive to make careful decisions about which cases to take. The attorney evaluates the prospective plaintiff's story, gauges the costs of bringing the lawsuit, and estimates the probability of success and the likely award *(15)*. If the contingency fee expected in the event of a win, discounted by the probability of losing, exceeds the expected litigation costs, then the attorney will take the case.

In summary, the functioning of the malpractice system is efficient in theory: the courts step in to compensate and deter where self-regulation has failed to prevent a breach of accepted standards of care; plaintiffs' attorneys serve as gatekeepers, separating meritorious from unpromising claims; and liability insurance ensures that providers are not bankrupted by a single large payout and resources are available to compensate patients. However, the actual operation of the system, as shown through its history and by empirical studies of litigation, presents a much more complicated story.

EVOLUTION OF MALPRACTICE LITIGATION

Despite several bursts of malpractice litigation in the 1800s *(16,17)*, suing physicians was an arduous undertaking until the latter half of the 20th century *(18,19)*. At that time, the judiciary began dismantling barriers that plaintiffs faced in bringing tort litigation *(20)*. This shift occurred in many areas of accident law, but it was particularly prominent in medical malpractice in the 1960s and early 1970s *(21,22)*. Judges discarded rules that had traditionally posed obstacles to litigation. For example, most jurisdictions rolled back charitable immunity for hospitals. Courts also moved toward national standards of care and abandoned strict interpretations of the locality rule, which had required plaintiffs to find expert witnesses within the defendant's immediate practice community *(18)*. At the same time, expansion of doctrines such as informed consent and *res ipsa loquitur* (the rule that events, like retained instruments after surgery, carry an inference of negligence) paved new pathways to the courtroom *(22)*. The more plaintiff-friendly environment fostered by these changes altered plaintiff attorneys' cost–benefit calculus, leading to steady growth in litigation.

The synergistic impact of changes in legal doctrine, advances in medical science, and the development of more coherent and visible standards of care eventually began to show in surges of litigation and plaintiff victories. By the mid-1970s, many states were facing a malpractice crisis, although the situation varied considerably from state to state *(23)*. Using data from the height of the crisis, Danzon identified a near 20-fold difference in claims rates and average payouts between low-activity states like Maine and a high-activity states like California and Nebraska *(24)*.

As claims and insurance premiums soared, major insurers exited the medical malpractice market, leaving many physicians without coverage. Health care institutions and insurers clamored for policy changes to degrease the wheels of litigation. State legislatures responded with a mix of tort reform measures. The exodus of insurers also forced several states to undertake insurance reform *(25)*: legislatures established quasi-public bodies called "joint underwriting associations" to serve as insurers of last resort *(18)*; special state patient compensation funds were introduced to absolve commercial insurers of responsibility for specified dollar portions of malpractice payments; and public reinsurance mechanisms were established to fill gaps in the underwriting market. By the late 1970s, the malpractice crisis had abated.

However, within several years, malpractice claims rates were climbing again, along with other types of personal injury litigation. The premium spikes of the mid-1980s touched virtually every state, prompting an even more comprehensive round of tort reform (25,26). Legislators were drawn especially to caps on noneconomic and punitive damages. The diffuse nature of this crisis meant that many of the reforms affecting malpractice cut widely across tort litigation (26). Calm returned by the end of the 1980s, but these successive crises wrought significant changes in the professional liability insurance industry. The historical market dominance of large property and casualty insurers was supplanted by the growth of institutional self-insurance arrangements and "bedpan mutuals," which are physician-owned and -managed insurance companies with medical malpractice as their sole line of business.

The 1990s saw little growth in claims rates and steady but generally manageable increases in average settlement amounts (28). Approximately 70% of claims closed with no payment, and defendants won the majority of cases that went to trial (29). Many insurers experienced favorable "loss ratios," the ratio of payments and administrative costs to premiums collected. Insurers had set premiums high, apprehensive that the troubles of the 1980s would continue, but, in fact, claims rates and payouts held relatively stable. In this favorable market, new entrants appeared, aggressively sought business from all newcomers, and set off fierce competition on premiums (30). As a result, premium growth was generally slow or nonexistent during this period. A distinct "insurance cycle" is thus apparent over the past quarter-century, in which trends in claiming, reinsurance costs, interest rates, and other factors cause premiums and insurer loss ratios to rise and fall over time (30,31).

EMPIRICAL RESEARCH ON THE FUNCTIONING OF THE MALPRACTICE SYSTEM

Until the 1970s, little was known about the epidemiology of medical malpractice or how well the system carried out its theoretical functions. In 1973, an influential government inquiry into medical malpractice (32) led to the first efforts to evaluate the system's efficacy from an epidemiologic perspective.

The Medical Insurance Feasibility Study (MIFS) undertook review of nearly 21,000 medical records from 23 California hospitals (33). The study found that 4.6% of hospitalizations involved iatrogenic injury and 0.8% (1 in 126 admissions) involved injuries that medicolegal experts thought would likely give rise to a finding of negligence in court *(33)*. Comparison of the negligent injuries to the frequency of malpractice claims in California showed a wide gulf: the former outstripped the latter by a factor of 10 *(24)*. This key finding provided an explanation for episodic increases in claims rates: the existence of a huge reservoir of injuries meant that plaintiff attorneys could initiate fewer or more claims at any given time, depending on their business decisions and the permissiveness of the legal environment.

Prompted by the malpractice crisis of the mid-1980s, a research team at Harvard University embarked on a review of medical records from more than 30,000 hospital discharges and 3500 malpractice claims in New York *(34)*. The reviewers found rates of adverse events and negligent adverse events (3.7% and 1%, respectively) that were remarkably close to those detected in California *(35)*. Extrapolations from these rates produced alarming estimates of the burden of medical injury, including projections that negligent care caused approx 20,000 disabling injuries and 7000 deaths in New York hospitals in 1984. Overall, there were 7.6 times more negligent injuries than claims.

However, it was the matching of specific claims to specific injuries in New York that threw the troubling relationship between malpractice claims and injuries into sharp relief. Only 2% of negligent injuries resulted in claims, and only 17% of claims appeared to involve a negligent injury *(36)*. Paul Weiler has analogized this relationship to a traffic cop who regularly gives out more tickets to drivers who go through green lights than to those who run red lights *(2)*. A third study conducted in Utah and Colorado in the late 1990s found injury rates similar to those from New York *(37)* and virtually identical disconnections between injury and litigation *(38)*, suggesting that the core problems were neither regionally nor temporally idiosyncratic.

Diagnoses of the system's capacity to compensate a valid claim once it has been filed are not as bleak. A number of studies have concluded that the tort system does a reasonably good job of directing compensation to plaintiffs with meritorious claims *(39–43)*. However, several other studies have shown fairly indiscriminate compensation of claims *(44,45)*, including a 10-year follow-up of the Harvard data from New York that found that the key predictor of payment was the plaintiff's degree of disability, not negligence *(45)*.

Regardless, the overall picture that emerges from these studies is disheartening. Using a wide lens—one that takes in all patients who experience negligent injury, not just those who manage to join the hunt for compensation as plaintiffs—the findings from California, New York, and Utah/Colorado are a searing indictment of the malpractice system's performance. The data reveal a profoundly inaccurate mechanism for distributing compensation. It is also a tremendously inefficient one: approx 60 cents of every dollar expended on the system is absorbed by administrative costs (predominantly on legal fees *[46]*), an amount is twice the overhead rate for an average workers' compensation scheme *(2)*.

There has been less empirical scrutiny of the malpractice system's performance as a deterrent of substandard care than there has been of its record as a compensation mechanism. Legal deterrence is a notoriously difficult phenomenon to measure *(47)*. A few studies have attempted to model the relationship between claims experience and subsequent adverse event rates, negligence rates, or quality-of-care indicators *(34,48,49)*. These studies have yielded mixed findings and are vulnerable to methodological criticism. Considered as a whole, the evidence that the system deters medical negligence can be characterized as limited at best *(50)*.

Ironically, some of the more convincing evidence that tort law influences provider behavior comes from several studies suggesting that it may do so in undesirable ways *(51–53)*—namely, by encouraging the ordering of tests and procedures that are of marginal or no medical benefit, primarily for the purpose of reducing medical-legal risk. The field of obstetrics has attracted the most thorough search for evidence of so-called defensive medicine. The picture is actually murkier than the conventional wisdom would suggest *(50)*. Several well-designed studies have found that higher malpractice risk increased the probability of delivery by Cesarean section *(51,52)*, others have found the opposite *(54)*, and still others have found no association *(49,55)*. The magnitude of the costs associated with defensive medicine is also uncertain. One analysis estimated system-wide costs to be in the range of $5 billion to $15 billion in 1991 dollars *(56)*, but the methods used in this study have been roundly criticized *(57)*, as have other estimates of the system-wide costs of defensive medicine *(58)*. In any case, defensive medicine remains a perennial issue in policy debates over the malpractice system *(50)*.

IS THE NEW CRISIS NEW?

The latest tort crisis is characterized by both the decreasing availability of insurance coverage, as insurers exit the market in response to deteriorating loss ratios, and decreasing affordability of policies offered by the remaining insurers. As we noted in an earlier report *(59)*, the genesis of the current crisis is best characterized as multifactorial. Three factors that have almost certainly played a role are: (a) dramatic increases in payouts to plaintiffs since 1999—a 60% increase in the average award (unadjusted for inflation) and a doubling of the percentage of payouts of $1 million or more during the 1997–2001 period, according to the Physician Insurers Association of America *(60)*; (b) moderate increases in the frequency of claims in some states *(31)*; and (c) the wider downturn in the economy, which tends to be reflected in lower stock values and bond interest rates, affecting insurers' investment returns *(30,31)*. Some also argue that imprudent business decisions by insurers during the 1990s have contributed to their present difficulties (e.g., growing their subscriber base too quickly and pricing premiums too low) *(31)*.

The causes of increases in claims frequency and severity are unclear, but plausible arguments can be made for at least five factors: (1) greater public awareness of medical error; (2) lower levels of patient confidence and trust following the negative experience with managed care; (3) advances in medical innovation, particularly diagnostic technology, and increases in the intensity of medical services *(61)*; (4) rising public expectations about medical care; and (5) a greater reluctance among plaintiffs' attorneys to accept offers that historically would have closed cases. The last factor may be explained in part by the first two factors if public skepticism about error has infiltrated jury attitudes and decision making.

As in past crises, the medical community asserts that it must adopt defensive practices to avoid lawsuits, such as ordering unnecessary tests and procedures and turning away high-risk cases *(57)*. A related claim is that rising insurance costs are endangering patient care by forcing physicians in high-risk specialties to leave practice or move to more hospitable jurisdictions and by forcing hospitals to close high-risk services such as obstetrics and emergency departments *(62)*. Plaintiff attorneys dispute the claims of compromised access and deny that defensive medicine imperils patient care; therefore, the malpractice debate at state and national levels proceeds along a well-worn path.

However, the familiar rancor should not lull observers into a sense of déjà vu. Two critical policy issues distinguish the current malpractice crisis from previous eras. First, the health care industry today has less capacity to absorb sudden increases in insurance premiums. In the 1980s, hospitals and physicians could generally pass a significant portion of such costs to payers *(63)*. The spread of managed care, the advent of strong price controls in Medicare (with very little adjustment, especially recently), and the widespread adoption of fee schedules by private insurers have lowered net incomes *(64)*, rendering physicians less able to cope with hikes in practice costs than in earlier tort crises.

Second, the present crisis occurs in the shadow of the new patient safety movement *(65)*. The Institute of Medicine's 2000 Report on medical error *(66)* galvanized public attention; almost overnight, it catapulted medical injury from a relatively obscure topic in health services research to the forefront of the nation's health policy agenda. Although the report skirted the topic of liability, the interconnectedness of patient safety and malpractice is increasingly apparent.

THE "TWO CULTURES" PROBLEM: MALPRACTICE LAW AND PATIENT SAFETY

The malpractice system lies in deep tension with the goals and initiatives of the patient safety movement. At root, there is a problem of two cultures *(67)*: trial attorneys believe that the threat of litigation makes doctors practice more safely, but tort law's punitive, individualistic, adversarial approach is antithetical to the nonpunitive, systems-oriented, cooperative strategies promoted by patient safety leaders.

For example, consider disclosure and reporting requirements. Transparency has become the leitmotif of patient safety movement. To learn from errors, we must first identify them; to identify them, we must foster an atmosphere conducive to openness about mistakes *(68)*. Hospitals and physicians are urged to be honest with patients about injury and medical error, to report such events to one another and to regulators, and to address methods of prevention openly *(69)*. To nurture openness, experts stress that most errors arise from proficient clinicians working in faulty systems, not from incompetence or carelessness *(66)*.

In sharp contrast, tort law targets individuals, assigning blame and compensation based on proof of negligence. Before, during, and after litigation, information about injuries and their surrounding circumstances is kept hidden. Risk-management activities typically are divorced from quality improvement *(70)*.

The clash between tort and patient safety cultures acts as a drag on efforts to improve quality. Concerns about malpractice exposure diminish the health care industry's appetite for patient safety activities *(71–73)*. The reluctance of physicians to buy into such activities stems from the perception that they are being asked to be open about errors with little or no assurance of legal protection at a time when litigation is on the rise, malpractice insurance is increasingly expensive and difficult to find, and claims history bears significantly on insurance prospects. This reluctance has manifested in several ways, but two of the most important are underreporting to adverse event reporting systems and chilled communication with patients about errors, especially preventable ones *(74,75)*.

Thus, in spite of malpractice law's mission to improve quality through deterrence—indeed, perhaps because of it—litigation fears obstruct progress in patient safety. The harsh reality is that greater publicity about mistakes, disclosure to patients, and access to reported information probably would increase litigation. Such corroborative information promises reduced time and costs for initiating litigation, shifting the plaintiff attorney's calculus in the direction of more lawsuits. Proponents of malpractice litigation applaud this, citing the prevalence of uncompensated negligent injuries and reiterating the importance of litigation as a deterrent. Critics are apprehensive and attempt to ensure that reporting systems are closed to the public. They may also seek to persuade providers that honest disclosure of errors actually decreases the probability of expensive litigation. Despite anecdotal reports of such positive experiences *(75,76)*, the notion that disclosure reduces litigation is largely unproven and somewhat implausible.

TORT REFORM

Each tort crisis has stimulated enthusiasm tort reform among policymakers. Conventional tort reforms divide roughly into three families (Table 1).

Reforms in the first family focus on limiting access to court. For example, screening panels force an evaluation of the merits of claims before they reach court. Their goal is to encourage settlement and stop nonmeritorious claims before they turn into protracted litigation. Another type of access constraint involves shortening statutes of limitation (time periods within which plaintiffs are permitted to sue after discovering their injury) or enacting statutes of repose (time limits that run from the date of the allegedly negligent event rather than discovery of the injury).

The second family of reforms modifies liability rules in an effort to reduce both the frequency of claims and the size of payouts. For example, eliminating joint-and-several liability means that a plaintiff may recover from multiple defendants only in proportion to their con-

Table 1
Malpractice Reform Options

Conventional tort reform		
Limitations on access to courts	*Modification of liability rules*	*Damages reform*
• Statute of limitations/ repose • Screening panels	• Joint and several liability rules • Informed consent • *Res ipsa loquitur*	• Caps • Attorney fee limits • Collateral source rules • Periodic payment
System reform		
Alternative mechanisms for resolving disputes	*Alternatives to negligence*	*Relocation of legal responsibility*
• Early offers • Medical courts • Private contracts • Fault-based administrative system	• "No-fault" administrative system • Predesignated compensable events	• Enterprise liability

tribution to causing the injury. Many states have enacted legislation reversing judicial expansions of liability *(77)*. Elimination of the doctrine of *res ipsa loquitur,* new standards for expert witnesses, and the imposition of higher standards for establishing breaches of informed consent all are examples of such retrenchment.

The third family of reforms directly addresses the size of awards, with caps on damages awards being by far the most prominent measure. The cap may be applied to the total damages award or only to the noneconomic (pain and suffering) component. More than half of the states already cap noneconomic damages, usually at ceilings ranging from $250,000 to $700,000 *(78)*. Caps enable insurers to better predict their exposure to losses. By making the most lucrative lawsuits worth less, damages caps also indirectly limit the contingency fee and ensure that fewer cases hold the promise of a favorable return on the attorney's investment. An alternative for achieving the same end is to limit the return itself through direct regulation of attorney fees, which is done in approximately one-third of the states.

Other tort reforms directed at reducing the size of awards include rules mandating "collateral source offsets" and "periodic payments." Collateral source offsets purport to stop plaintiffs from double-dipping by denying compensation for losses that may be recouped from other sources, such as health insurance. "Periodic payments" mean that total awards are not paid in lump sum; instead, plaintiffs receive the part of the award that covers future losses in installments as the expenditures arise.

It is too soon to judge the impact of the most recent wave of reforms, but studies from earlier eras are informative. Regression analyses *(25,79–82)* controlling for the presence of multiple tort reforms in a state, along with other characteristics of states or claims, have found that damages caps significantly reduce payouts (Table 2), but their impact on premiums is less clear. (Premium levels are responsive to various factors beside litigation dynamics, including previous losses, expected investment returns, business strategy, and the requirement in most states to gain approval from insurance regulators for rate changes *[31]*.) Several of these studies found that collateral source offsets reduce payouts and claim frequency but not premiums. In some analyses, shorter statutes of limitation appear to impact claim frequency and insurance premiums. Pretrial screening panels, binding arbitration, and regulation of attorney fees generally do not have significant impacts (Table 2). One study showed that insurers' loss ratios improved after caps were adapted *(82a)*, whereas another showed no significant effect *(82b)*. In addition, one recent study found that the presence of damages caps in a state is associated with higher growth in the supply of physicians over time *(83)*.

Critics of malpractice litigation frequently point out that it is very unrealistic to expect that increased levels of malpractice litigation will promote patient safety or make injury compensation more accurate or fair. The weight of empirical evidence supports this charge. However, often lost in the current debate is the recognition that it is every bit as unrealistic to expect that decreasing the number of lawsuits or the size of damages awards, which are the aims of conventional tort reform, will achieve these goals. Some conventional tort reforms appear to be effective in reducing litigation costs and stabilizing insurance markets, but they are not designed to remedy the fundamental failings of the malpractice system, nor will they. That objective requires more sweeping reform.

SYSTEM REFORM

Since the 1980s, a growing sense that the tort system is broken has prompted formulation of a number of alternatives for achieving compensation and deterrence. The leading recommendations, shown in the lower half of Table 1, are divided roughly into three approaches: (1)

Table 2
Study Findings: Impact of Tort Reforms of 1970s and Early 1980s

	Decrease claim payouts?	Decrease claim frequency?	Lower liability insurance premiums?
Damages cap (noneconomic or total)	Significant in three of four studies.	NS in the only study.	NS in two of two studies.
Collateral source offset	Significant in two of four studies.	Significant in one of two studies.	NS in two of two studies.
Pretrial screening panels	NS in four of four studies.	NS in three of three studies.	Significant in one of two studies.
Shorter statute of limitations	NS in two of three studies.	Significant in two of three studies.	Significant in one of two studies.
Binding arbitration	NS in two of three studies.	NS in three of three studies.	NS in two of two studies.
Attorney fee limits	NS in four of four studies.	NS in the only study.	NS in two of two studies.

NS, not significant. (Data from refs. 25,79–82.)

use of alternative mechanisms to resolve disputes; (2) dispensing with the negligence as the basis for compensation ("no-fault"); and (3) locating responsibility for accidents at the institutional level ("enterprise liability").

The alternative to litigation that is enjoying widest interest at the moment is an "Early Offer" program in which patients and the health care organization would have incentives to negotiate private settlements immediately after an adverse event occurs *(84–86)*. Other proposals would route malpractice claims through structured mediation *(87)*, administrative law hearings *(88)*, or medical courts *(89,90)*. Several scholars have also paired alternative mechanisms for resolving disputes with an emphasis on private contracts, allowing patients to agree in advance with their provider or health plan to submit to specified procedures, such as arbitration, in the event of an injury *(91–93)*.

A more radical approach to system reform would emulate workers' compensation and remove negligence as the basis of eligibility for compensation *(94)*. One version of this approach would empower an administrative agency to judge compensation for all medical injury claims *(95)*; another version would carve out from the tort system only certain classes of events—clinical outcomes that, by their very nature, are likely to have been preventable—and fast track them for adjudication according to predefined compensation criteria *(96,97)*.

The no-fault label traditionally given to this class of proposals is misleading because, following the lead of other countries, most actually replace the negligence determination with one of avoidability *(98,99)*. An avoidability standard is more permissive than negligence. For example, bleeding following a limited colectomy that necessitates reoperation, more significant resection of the bowel, and ileostomy would always be considered avoidable, but determining whether this event is negligent would likely require careful review of the facts of the surgery. Because avoidability criteria make a larger pool of injuries eligible for compensation, they trigger cost concerns *(99)*. Proponents contend that other efficiencies, such as reduced administrative and legal costs, should allay budgetary concerns; emphasize the prospects of fairer, more efficient compensation; and tout the close fit between the concept of avoidability and the system's focus of the patient safety movement as a major strength *(73)*.

Finally, a number of commentators have proposed establishing hospitals or integrated delivery systems as the sole locus of legal responsibility *(100,101)*. In so-called enterprise liability models, the enterprise assumes primary responsibility for any claim brought against an affiliated clinician and covers affiliates' liability costs at rates that vary from year to year according to the enterprise's overall injury experience. It is argued that an organizational approach to compensation and deterrence along these lines would underscore the value of systemic approaches to quality improvement *(85)*.

Sweeping system reforms, such as administrative compensation schemes and enterprise liability, have attracted some high-profile support in the current debate. Both the Institute of Medicine *(85)* and the blue-ribbon Governor's Select Task Force on Healthcare Professional Liability Insurance in Florida *(102)* have endorsed pilot projects. However, it seems politically unlikely that any of the most powerful voices in the debate will step forward to champion such initiatives. Organized medicine and the insurance industry continue to push for conventional tort reform and welcome the Bush Administration's focus on damages caps. The trial bar, a powerful constituency for the Democratic Party, is focused on scuttling this reform and can be expected to resist vigorously any attempt at fundamental system change.

A more likely scenario is that the current enthusiasm for change will result in another round of conventional tort reform, perhaps supplemented by federal legislation that includes one or two innovative but modest system reforms, such as an Early Offer Program. This may have some beneficial impacts on insurance markets over the medium to long term. Unfortunately, it will do little to alleviate the haphazardness of compensation for patients injured by medical care, and those interested in advancing patient safety will continue to wrestle with an adversarial litigation system that undermines aspirations of transparency and error reduction. Remediation of these more fundamental shortcomings requires more fundamental reform.

ACKNOWLEDGMENT

This chapter is reprinted with permission from Studdert DM, Mello MM, Brennan TA. Medical malpractice. N Engl J Med. 2004; 350(3):283–292. (Copyright © 2004 Massachusetts Medical Society. All rights reserved.)

REFERENCES

1. O'Connell J. The lawsuit lottery: only the lawyers win. New York, NY: Free Press, 1979.
2. Weiler PC, Hiatt HH, Newhouse JP, Johnson WG, Brennan T, Leape LL. A measure of malpractice: medical injury, malpractice litigation, and patient compensation. Cambridge, MA: Harvard University Press, 1993.

3. Boyle LV. The truth about medical malpractice. Trial, April, 2002. (*see* Website: http://www.atla.org/medmal/prez.aspx. Last accessed, July 2003)

4. Keeton WP, Dobbs DB, Keeton RE, Owens DG. Prosser & Keeton on the Law of Torts. 5th Ed. St. Paul, MN: West Publishing Co., 1984.

5. Mello MM. Of Swords and Shields: The use of clinical practice guidelines in medical malpractice litigation. Univ Penn Law Rev 2000;149(3):645–710.

6. Hyams AL, Shapiro DW, Brennan TA. Medical practice guidelines in malpractice litigation: an early retrospective. J Health Polit Policy Law. 1996;21(2):289–313.

7. Peters PG. The role of the jury in modern malpractice law. Iowa Law Rev 2002:909–969.

8. Shavell S. Economic analysis of accident law. Cambridge, MA: Harvard University Press, 1987.

9. Calabresi G. The cost of accidents: a legal and economic analysis. New Haven, CT: Yale University Press, 1970.

10. Schwartz WB, Mendelson DN. Physicians who have lost their malpractice insurance: their demographic characteristics and the surplus-line companies that insure them. JAMA 1989;262:1335–1341.

11. Hickson GB, Clayton EW, Entman SS, et al. Obstetricians' prior malpractice experience and patients' satisfaction with care. JAMA 1994;272:1583–1587.

12. Hickson GB, Federspiel CF, Pichert JW, et al. Patient complaints and malpractice risk. JAMA. 2002;287:2951–2957.

13. Levinson W, Roter DL, Mullooly JP, Dull VT, Frankel RM. Physician-patient communication. The relationship with malpractice claims among primary care physicians and surgeons. JAMA 1997;277:553–559.

14. Hickson GB, Clayton EW, Githens PB. Factors that prompted families to file medical malpractice claims following perinatal injuries. JAMA 1992;268: 1413–1414.

15. Kritzer HK. The justice broker: lawyers and ordinary litigation. New York, NY: Oxford Univ. Press, 1990.

16. DeVille KA. Medical Malpractice in Nineteenth-Century America: Origins and Legacy. New York, NY: New York University Press, 1990.

17. Mohr JC. American medical malpractice litigation in historical perspective. JAMA. 2000;283:1731–1737.

18. Weiler PC. Medical Malpractice on Trial. Cambridge, MA: Harvard University Press, 1991.

19. Opinion survey on medical professional liability. JAMA 1957;164:1583–1594.

20. Rabin RL (ed). Perspectives on Tort Law, 4th Ed. Boston, MA: Little Brown, 1995.

21. Schwartz GT. Medical malpractice, tort, contract, and managed care. Univ Illinois Law Rev. 1998;1998:885–907.

22. Havighurst CC, Blumstein JF, Brennan TA. Health care law and policy: readings, notes, and questions. 2nd Ed. New York, NY: Foundation Press, 1998.

23. Robinson GO. The medical malpractice crisis of the 1970s: a retrospective. Law and Contemp Probs 1986;49:5–36.

24. Danzon PM. Medical malpractice: theory, evidence and public policy. Cambridge, MA: Harvard University Press, 1985.

25. Sloan, FA. State responses to the malpractice insurance "crisis" of the 1970s: an empirical assessment. J Health Polit Pol Law 1985;9:629–645.

26. Bovbjerg RR. Legislation on medical malpractice: further developments and a preliminary report card. UC Davis Law Rev 1989;22:499–566.
27. Kinney, ED, Malpractice reform in the 1990s: past disappointments, future success? J Health Polit Pol Law 1995;20:99–136.
28. Studdert DM, Brennan TA, Thomas EJ. Beyond dead reckoning: Measures of medical injury burden, malpractice litigation, and alternative compensation models from Utah and Colorado. Indiana Law Rev 2000;33:1643–1686.
29. Physician Insurers Association of America. Data Sharing Project Information Manual. Rockville, MD, 2001.
30. Bovbjerg RR, Bartow A. Understanding Pennsylvania's Medical Malpractice Crisis. (*see* Website:http//www.medliabilitypa.org/research/report0603/Under standingReport.pdf. Last accessed July 2003).
31. United States General Accounting Office, Medical malpractice insurance: multiple factors have contributed to increased premium rates. GAO-03-702. Washington, DC: GAO, June 2003.
32. United States Department of Health, Education and Welfare. Medical malpractice: Report of the Secretary's Commission on Medical Malpractice DHEW Publication No. (OS) 73–89. Washington, DC: DHES, 1973.
33. Mills DH (ed). California Medical Association and California Hospital Association Report on the Medical Insurance Feasibility Study. San Francisco, CA: Sutter Publications 1977.
34. Harvard Medical Practice Study Investigators. Patients, doctors, and lawyers: medical injury, malpractice litigation, and patient compensation in New York. Report of the Harvard Medical Practice Study to the state of New York. Cambridge, MA: The President and Fellows of Harvard College, 1990.
35. Brennan TA, Leape LL, Laird NM, et al. Incidence of adverse events and negligence in hospitalized patients. Results of the Harvard Medical Practice Study I. New Engl J Med 1991;324:370–376.
36. Localio AR, Lawthers AG, Brennan TA, et al. Relation between malpractice claims and adverse events due to negligence. Results of the Harvard Medical Practice Study III. N Engl J Med. 1991;325(4):245–251.
37. Thomas EJ, Studdert DM, Burstin HR, et al. Incidence and risk factors for adverse events and negligent care in Utah and Colorado in 1992. Med Care 2000;38:261–271.
38. Studdert DM, Thomas EJ, Burstin HR, Zbar BI, Orav EJ, Brennan TA. Negligent care and malpractice claiming behavior in Utah and Colorado. Med Care 2000;38:250–260.
39. Taragin MI, Willett LR, Wilczek AP, Trout R, Carson JL. The influence of standard of care and severity of injury on the resolution of medical malpractice claims. Ann Intern Med 1992;117:780–784.
40. Vidmar N. Medical malpractice and the American jury: confronting the myths about jury incompetence, deep pockets, and outrageous damage awards. Ann Arbor, MI: University of Michigan Press, 1995.
41. Sloan FA, Hsieh CR. Variability in medical malpractice payments: is the compensation fair? Law Soc Rev 1990;24:997–1039.
42. White MJ. The value of liability in medical malpractice. Health Aff 1994;13:75–87.
43. Sloan FA, Githens PB, Clayton EW, Hickson GB, Gentile DA, Partlett DF. Suing for medical malpractice. Chicago, IL: Univ Chic Press, 1993.

44. Cheney FW, Posner K, Caplan RA, Ward RJ: Standard of care and anesthesia liability. JAMA 1989;261:1599–1603.
45. Brennan TA, Sox CA, Burstin HR. Relation between negligent adverse events and the outcomes of medical malpractice litigation. New Engl J Med. 1996;335: 1963–1967.
46. Kakalik JS, Pace NM. Costs and compensation paid in tort litigation. R-3391-ICJ. Santa Monica, CA: RAND, 1986.
47. Schwartz GT. Reality in the economic analysis of tort law: does tort law really deter? UCLA L Rev 1994;42:377–444.
48. Entman SS, Glass CA, Hickson GB, Githens PB, Whetten-Goldstein K, Sloan FA. Relationship between malpractice claims history and subsequent obstetric care. JAMA 1994;272:1588–1591.
49. Sloan FA, Whetten-Goldstein K, Githens PB, Entman SS. Effects of the threat of medical malpractice litigation and other factors on birth outcomes. Med Care 1995;33:700–714.
50. Mello MM, Brennan TA. Deterrence of medical errors: theory and evidence for malpractice reform. Tex Law Rev. 2002;80:1595–1637.
51. Dubay L, Kaestner R, Waidmann T. The impact of malpractice fears on cesarean section rates. J Health Econ 1999;18(4):491–522.
52. Localio AR, Lawthers AG, Bengtson JM, et al. Relationship between malpractice claims and cesarean delivery. JAMA 1993; 269(3):366–373.
53. Kessler D, McClellan M. Do doctors practice defensive medicine? Q J Econ 1996;111:353-390.
54. Tussing DA, Wojtowycz MA. The cesarean decision in New York state, 1986: economic and noneconomic aspects. Med Care 1992;30:529–540.
55. Baldwin L, Hart LG, Lloyd M, et al. Defensive medicine and obstetrics. JAMA 1995;274:1606–1610.
56. Rubin R, Mendelson DJ. How much does defensive medicine cost? J Am Health Pol 1994;4:7–15.
57. US Congress, Office of Technology Assessment. Defensive medicine and medical malpractice. OTA-H-602. Washington, DC: Government Printing Office, 1994.
58. General Accounting Office. Medical malpractice: implications of rising premiums on access to health care. GAO-03-836. Washington, DC: General Accounting Office, August 2003.
59. Mello MM, Studdert DM, Brennan TA. The new medical malpractice crisis. New Engl J Med 2003;348:2281–2284.
60. Physician Insurers Association of America. Statement by the Physician Insurers Association of America, January 29, 2003. (*see* Website: http//www.thepiaa.org/pdf_files/january_29_piaa_statement.pdf2003. Last accessed, July 2003)
61. Sage WM. Understanding the first malpractice crisis of the 21st century. In Gosfield AG (ed.) Health law handbook. St. Paul, MN: West Group, 2003 (in press).
62. Palmisano DJ. Statement of the American Medical Association to the Committee on Energy and Commerce, Subcommittee on Health, U.S. House of Representatives Re: Assessing the Need to Enact Medical Liability Reform. Feb. 27, 2003. (*see* Website: http://www.ama-assn.org/ama/pub/article/6281-7334.html. Last accessed July 2003)
63. Danzon PM, Pauly MV, Kington RS. The effects of malpractice litigation on physicians' fees and incomes. Amer Econ Rev 1990;80:122–127.

64. Reed M, Ginsburg PB. Behind the times: physician income, 1995-99. Data Bull (Cent Stud Health Syst Change) 2003;24:1–2.
65. Sage WM. Medical liability and patient safety. Health Aff 2003;22(4):26–36.
66. Corrigan J, Donaldson M (eds). To err is human: building a safer health system. Washington, DC: Institute of Medicine, 2000.
67. Bovbjerg RR, Miller RH, Shapiro DW. Paths to reducing medical injury: Professional liability and discipline vs. patient safety—and the need for a third way. J Law Med Ethics 200 Fall-Winter;29:369–380.
68. Reason J. Human error: models and management. Brit Med J 2000;320:768–770.
69. Berwick DM, Leape LL. Reducing errors in medicine: it's time to take this more seriously. Brit Med J 1999; 319:136–137.
70. Morlock LL, Lindgren OH, Cassirer C, Mills DH. Medical liability and clinical risk management. In Goldfield N, Nash D (eds.). Managing quality of care in a cost-focused environment. Tampa, FL: American College of Physician Executives, 1999.
71. Liang BA. Risks of reporting sentinel events. Health Aff. 2000;19(5):112–120.
72. Gostin LO. A public health approach to reducing error: medical malpractice as a barrier. JAMA 2000;283:1742–1743.
73. Studdert DM, Brennan TA. No-fault compensation for medical injuries: the prospect for error prevention. JAMA 2001;286:217–223.
74. Blendon RJ, DesRoches CM, Brodie M, Benson JM, Rosen AB, Schneider E, et al. Views of practicing physicians and the public on medical errors. New Engl J Med 2002;347:1933–1940.
75. Lamb RM, Studdert DM, Bohmer RMJ, Berwick DM, Brennan TA. Hospital disclosure practices: results of a national survey. Health Aff 2003(2);22: 73–83.
76. Kraman SS, Hamm G. Risk management: extreme honesty may be the best policy. Ann Intern Med 1999;131:963–967.
77. Rustad ML, Koenig TH. Taming the monster: the American civil justice system as a battleground for social theory. Brooklyn Law Rev 2002;68:1–105.
78. National Conference of State Legislatures. State medical liability laws table (see Website: http://www.ncsl.org/programs/insur/medliability.pdf. Last accessed July, 2002).
79. Danzon P. The frequency and severity of medical malpractice claims. J Law Econ 1984;27:115–148.
80. Danzon PM. The frequency and severity of medical malpractice claims: new evidence. Law Contemp Probs 1986;49:57–84.
81. Sloan FA, Mergenhagen PM, Bovbjerg RR. Effects of tort reforms on the value of closed medical malpractice claims: a microanalysis. J Health Polit Pol Law 1989;14:663–689.
82. Zuckerman S, Bovbjerg RR, Sloan F. Effects of tort reforms and other factors on medical malpractice insurance premiums. Inquiry 1990;27:167–182.
82a. Born PH, Viscusi WK. The distribution of the insurance market effects of tort liability reforms. In: Brookings papers on economic activity: microeconomics. Washington DC: Brookings Institute 1998;55:105.
82b. Viscusi WK, Zeckhauser RJ, Born PH, Blackman G. The effect of 1980s tort reform legislation on general liability and medical malpractice insurance. J Risk Uncertain 1993;6:165–186.

83. Hellinger FJ, Encinosa WE. The impact of state laws limiting malpractice awards on the geographic distribution of physicians. U.S. Department of Health and Human Services, Agency for Healthcare Research and Quality, Center for Organization and Delivery Studies. July 3, 2003.
84. Office of the Assistant Secretary for Planning and Evaluation, Department of Health and Human Services. Addressing the new health care crisis: reforming the medical litigation system to improve the quality of health care. March 3, 2003.
85. Corrigan J, Greiner A, Erickson SM (eds). Fostering rapid advances in health care: learning from system demonstrations. Washington, DC: Institute of Medicine, 2002.
86. O'Connell J. Offers that can't be refused: foreclosure of personal injury claims by defendants' prompt tender of claimants' net economic losses. Northwestern Law Rev 1982;77:589–632.
87. Dauer EA, Marcus LJ. Adapting mediation to link resolution of medical malrpactice disputes with health care quality improvement. Law Contemp Prob 1997;60(1):185–218.
88. Jonson KB, Phillips CG, Orentlicher D, Hatlie MS. A fault-based administrative alternative for resolving medical malpractice claims. Vand Law Rev 1989;42: 1365–1406.
89. Howard PK. The best course of treatment. New York Times. July 21, 2003:A15.
90. S. 1518. Reliable Medical Justice Act. 108th Congress, 2003.
91. Epstein RA. Medical malpractice: the case for contract. Am Bar Found Res J 1976:87–149.
92. O'Connell J. Neo-no-fault remedies for medical injuries: coordinated statutory and contractual alternatives. Law Contemp Prob 1986 Spring;49:125–141.
93. Havighurst CC. Health Care Choices: Private contracts as instruments of health reform. Washington, DC: AEI Press, 1995.
94. Bovbjerg RR, Sloan FA. No-fault for medical injury: theory and evidence. U Cincinnati Law Rev 1998;67:53–123.
95. Weiler PC. The case for no-fault medical liability. Maryland Law Rev 1993;52:908–950.
96. Havighurst CC, Tancredi LR. Medical adversity insurance—a no-fault approach to medical malpractice and quality assurance. Milb Mem Fund Quart 1974;51: 125–168.
97. Bovbjerg RR, Tancredi LR, Gaylin DS. Obstetrics and malpractice: evidence on the performance of a selective no-fault system. JAMA 1991;265:2836–2843.
98. Danzon PM. The Swedish patient compensation system: lessons for the United States. J Leg Med 1994;15:199–248.
99. Studdert DM, Thomas EJ, Zbar BI, Newhouse JP, Weiler PC, Brennan TA. Can the United States afford a no-fault system of compensation for medical injury? Law Contemp Probs 1997;60:1–34.
100. Abraham KS, Weiler PC. Enterprise medical liability and the evolution of the American health care system. Harv Law Rev. 1994;108:381–436.
101. Sage WM, Hastings KE, Berenson RA. Enterprise liability for medical malpractice and health care quality improvement. Am J Law Med. 1994;10(1&2):1–28.
102. Florida Governor's Select Task Force on Healthcare Professional Liability Insurance. Report and Recommendations. Tallahassee, FL: Office of the Governor, 2003.

17 New Directions in Medical Liability Reform

William M. Sage, MD, JD

SUMMARY

Medical malpractice is the "Rip van Winkle" issue in American health care. However, its periodic awakenings depart from those of its fictional counterpart in an important respect. Neither the participants in the medical malpractice system nor outside observers seem aware that the context for minimizing medical errors, improving legal dispute resolution, and keeping liability insurance available and affordable has changed. This chapter explains why the public policy of medical malpractice is so poorly connected to overall health policy. It examines three aspects of health system change since the 1970s—medical progress, industrialization, and cost containment—that have exposed serious weaknesses in the medical liability system. It suggests ways to convert liability into a general health policy issue, including having the federal government implement a system of error identification, fair compensation, and efficient dispute resolution that would apply to Medicare and Medicaid patients.

Key Words: Medical malpractice; tort liability; medical technology; health insurance; Medicare; managed care; patient safety; medical errors; litigation; liability insurance.

From: *Medical Malpractice: A Physician's Sourcebook*
Edited by: R. E. Anderson © Humana Press Inc., Totowa, NJ

MALPRACTICE RESURRECTED

Medical malpractice is the Rip van Winkle of the health care system. In 2002, liability insurance premiums rose suddenly from their stupor after slumbering—sometimes peacefully, sometimes fitfully—for nearly two decades. Much as Washington Irving's hero found his physical surroundings unlike those he remembered, today's malpractice system faces a landscape of health care financing and delivery that has changed much since its last awakening. Rip van Winkle slept through the American revolution, and the intervening years between the last malpractice crisis and the present one have witnessed equally dramatic changes wrought by medical technology, consumer demand, managed care, and Medicare cost containment. Unlike its fictional counterpart, however, the malpractice system does not strike most observers as anachronistic. When Rip van Winkle wandered down from the hills, the townspeople noticed immediately that his musket was antiquated and his clothes were outdated. This is not so for medical liability, although it has been largely out of sight and out of mind (at least for physicians) since the 1980s. With few exceptions, stakeholders and their political allies on both sides of the tort reform debate invoke the same explanations and propose the same legislation as they did 20 years ago: measures discouraging lawsuits and limiting damage awards that are at best incomplete and at worst obsolete.

To switch metaphors, several commentators have described the current liability insurance crisis as a "perfect storm." Indeed, an unprecedented confluence of forces has contributed to rising premiums for health care providers in many specialties and many parts of the country. These include large jury awards and settlements, harsh economic conditions that reduce returns on funds invested by liability insurers, a spate of pull-outs and insolvencies among carriers, and a series of catastrophes unrelated to health care that have caused a global contraction in reinsurance capital. However, sailors in the right vessel using proper tactics can ride out even the most severe weather. A properly designed liability system that reduces the incidence of medical error, limits unnecessary monetary and psychic costs associated with redressing injury, and bears residual insurance risk efficiently would have much greater resilience in troughs of the insurance cycle than the structures and processes currently being used. Unfortunately, the storm analogy—which is used to convey the gravity of the current predicament—carries with it a sense of helplessness as well. Therefore, most malpractice reform proposals at most try to steer flimsy craft into (hopefully) calmer waters. Relatively little attention is paid to re-engineering the system to survive harsh conditions, although forecasts for the future remain rather bleak.

In other words, time and tide have changed both the medical malpractice problem and its range of potential solutions. Yet the evolution of the health care system since the malpractice crisis of the 1980s has gone unrecognized by policymakers and partisans where liability is concerned.

Doctors and Lawyers

One can identify several possible explanations for the failure of the political process to integrate liability policy with overall health policy. From the perspective of doctors and lawyers—the key stakeholders in the continuing battle over tort reform—the implications of changing the health system muddy the "message" of their campaigns. As the health care system becomes more complex, so too does the liability system. Because the added complexity does not cut clearly in favor of or against measures such as caps on noneconomic damages, neither side gains advantage by addressing it. In addition, the current heads of professional associations on both sides (i.e., physicians and plaintiff attorneys) are frequently individuals who were drawn into "organized" medicine or law during earlier periods of crisis and slowly worked their way up through the ranks to leadership positions in local, state, and eventually national organizations. It is not surprising that many of them see the current crisis through the lens of their earlier experiences or that they attach great importance to winning the unfinished battles of their youths.

Government Structure

For health care regulators, medical liability remains *sui generis*. The inherent power of the judicial branch of government to dictate civil procedure, coupled with decentralization and lack of transparency in the private litigation process, segregates liability from other health regulatory concerns and gives it a distinctly "legal" flavor that discomfits nonlawyer bureaucrats. Health policy is also made at the federal level to a larger extent now than in 1975 or 1985, whereas malpractice is still primarily a creature of state law. In many respects, Medicare policy has become health policy, and liability issues are essentially invisible in Medicare and other federal health programs.

Politics

For federal and state legislators and the political parties they represent, medical liability is a reliable source of campaign contributions, giving them a vested interest both in continuing the contest and in divorcing liability from other health care issues. The longstanding nature of the legislative standoff has bred specialization among lobbyists for the key organizations, which often is reinforced by legislative rules vesting jurisdiction over civil litigation in judiciary committees that handle few other health care matters. Most significantly, the political importance of medical malpractice reform extends far beyond its impact on the health care system. One of the largest political questions under active debate in the United States deals with how personal injury lawsuits affect our economy and our social fabric. Business interests, corporate law firms, and the Republican Party view personal injury claims as costly and destructive, whereas organized consumer interests, the trial bar, and the Democratic Party consider recourse to litigation a last line of defense for individual rights in postindustrial society. Because of its emotional resonance with voters and its grassroots constituencies, malpractice reform is an attractive "poster child" for (and sometimes against) general tort reform. When malpractice premiums rise rapidly (as they are rising now), tort reformers bottle physician anguish for sale to the voting public. When premiums are stable, tort supporters try to peel physicians (and their patients) away from large business interests, as occurred during the decade-long debate over the right to sue HMOs for physical injury as part of a federal "patient protection act."

Research

Finally, both researchers and research sponsors go where the action is. Accordingly, most of what we know about the malpractice system derives from studies conducted during the crises of the 1970s and 1980s. In many cases, these findings have radically altered policy experts' understanding of the malpractice system. Ironically, the political stakeholders remain fixated on reform proposals from the 1970s and 1980s although sound empirical studies have dispelled some of the myths on which those reforms were predicated. On the other hand, little empirical investigation of medical liability tends to occur during the longer intervening stretches between crises. Like its predecessors, the current crisis has prompted a flurry of research activity, but the results of the most objective and comprehensive studies may not be available until after the acute phase of the crisis subsides. Therefore, policymakers seeking to take immediate action must interpret older data in light of known changes to the health care system since the last crisis occurred more than 15 years ago.

LIABILITY AND HEALTH SYSTEM CHANGE

Although the notion that physicians owe a legal duty of competence to patients extends back hundreds of years, its connection to public policy is of more recent vintage and is closely linked to two related phenomena: (a) the transformation of health care from a personal service to a complex series of industrial processes, and (b) its simultaneous recognition as a public resource heavily funded and heavily regulated by government. The malpractice crisis that began in 2002 can best be understood as a product of these changes. The principal lesson to be learned from this analysis is that the current crisis reflects the successes of modern medicine far more than it reflects the failures. As medical science improves, the opportunity cost of mistreatment rises. As health care delivery becomes more complicated, sources of error multiply. As medical expenditures grow, public and private payers manage them by intruding, directly and indirectly, on the prerogatives of health care providers. All of these trends magnify the risk of malpractice litigation and the cost of resolving it.

Medical Progress

Historically, no factor has driven malpractice risk more than medical progress. The first wave of malpractice suits in the mid-19th century alleged that fractures of long bones had been set improperly; a decade earlier, the standard of care had been to amputate *(1,2)*. Since that time, every addition to the scientific capabilities of medicine has been accompanied by rising public expectations, which translates to a heightened legal standard of care and greater willingness on the part of judges and juries to attribute poor outcomes to misadventure rather than misfortune *(3)*. Parallel improvements in diagnostic and therapeutic modalities make omissions an increasingly important source of litigation, with brief delays in diagnosis arguably causing measurable injury even in frail and elderly patients. Medical progress also implies greater need for monetary compensation, primarily to fund increasingly expensive and prolonged treatment for iatrogenic injury. For this reason, long-term trends in the aggregate cost of malpractice insurance closely track growth in national health care expenditures.

A Texas case decided in 2002 offers a representative example of how health system change has altered the nature of both medical error and malpractice compensation. In *Brownsville Pediatric Association v. Reyes*, 68 S.W.3d 184 (Tex. App. 2002), the court upheld a jury award of $8 million to a child suffering from blindness and spastic paraplegia.

The child had been born prematurely and allegedly had been injured while receiving care in a neonatal intensive care unit. The allegations of substandard care related mainly to intubation, mechanical ventilation, and exchange transfusion. The court estimated the child's life expectancy at 53 years and awarded $6.5 million to defray future medical expenses. The most costly element of future care was an implantable pump that would infuse a novel drug directly into the spinal canal to reduce spasticity. Twenty-five years ago, fewer premature infants survived, life expectancies for children with severe injuries were shorter, and medications that can now be given to improve function were not available.

Industrialization

A more successful health care system is necessarily more industrialized. Although the relationship between patient and physician remains important to both technical and interpersonal quality, delivering health care requires coordinating an array of individual and institutional services and providing manufactured items that range from pharmaceuticals to durable medical equipment. The cost of health care in the United States exceeds $1.5 trillion annually and can only be sustained through sophisticated financing mechanisms for both personal health insurance and industrial capital formation *(4)*. Not surprisingly, the professional and charitable underpinnings of the medical enterprise have been supplemented, if not wholly supplanted, by commercial activity.

Malpractice insurance crises are the exception, not the rule. During the much longer periods of relative stability between crises, industrialization in health care (as in society in general) has been accompanied by a steady expansion of liability. Specialization raised the bar for physician practice and reduced application of the locality rule. Doctrines of charitable immunity that once protected hospitals eroded as patients obtained insurance and became paying customers. As their capital resources grew, institutional providers also came under more pressure from tort law to ensure the availability of medical technology than had typically been applied to individual physicians and faced closer scrutiny regarding possible financial motives for failing to render optimal care. As discussed below, these trends are problematic when malpractice crises strike because physicians' share of medical liability persistently exceeds their proportionate share of industrial revenue and, therefore, risk-bearing capacity. Furthermore, corporate health care providers such as managed care organizations (and hospitals acting as competitive enterprises) face a higher risk of punitive damages than individual physicians *(5)*.

Cost Containment

The malpractice crises of the 1970s and 1980s hit during the best of times (at least financially) for physicians and hospitals. The decades from World War II through the implementation of Medicare are generally considered American medicine's "golden age." Faith in the beneficial potential of health care generated massive financial investments from both public and private sources, which were placed under the unfettered control of physicians. Dramatic increases in malpractice litigation toward the end of this period arguably sought to justify the public's trust. Lawsuits imposed real emotional and reputational costs on defendants but seldom constituted a severe financial burden. As studies from the 1980s demonstrated, even substantial increases in liability insurance premiums were quickly passed through to patients and payers as higher fees *(6,7)*.

By contrast, the current malpractice crisis follows nearly two decades of sustained effort to rein in health care spending. Cost-based reimbursement and "usual and customary" fees are, in most cases, distant memories. Medicare pays administrative prices that are not responsive to unexpected jumps in short-term input costs for providers. Private health insurers are equally reluctant to renegotiate provider contracts. Lack of these safety valves potentially impairs access to care for patients in already underserved communities if hospitals or physicians find liability insurance unaffordable. Even in areas where the supply of physicians and hospitals remains high, the health care system is less financially resilient and a malpractice crisis can seriously disrupt medical careers and therapeutic relationships.

Cost containment has also had important direct effects on malpractice exposure and on physicians' reactions to it. Higher throughput to maintain revenue, greater delegation of tasks to nonprofessional staff, and complex administrative systems of managed care oversight all increase risk of error, and the undercurrent of financial motivation makes patients less trusting and more litigious. Against this backdrop of cost-containment, a widening malpractice crisis epitomizes physicians' growing sense that they have lost control over their professional lives. This strikes physicians as particularly unfair because tort law still attributes to them a much higher degree of clinical autonomy and authority than their day-to-day experiences suggest.

Table 1
Five Major Problems of the Malpractice System

1. Compensation to patients for avoidable injury is inadequate.
2. Too many avoidable medical errors occur.
3. The litigation process is too slow, too costly, too uncertain, and too unpleasant.
4. Premiums for primary liability coverage are too volatile and, for some physicians, too expensive.
5. Excess coverage and reinsurance are becoming unaffordable for hospitals and other medical institutions.

EXPOSED WEAKNESSES IN THE MALPRACTICE SYSTEM

The pressures described in the preceding section have exposed major weaknesses in the way that allegations of medical malpractice are handled. Much like the American health care system itself, the malpractice system is a patchwork of historically derived institutions and practices rather than a product of careful deliberation or rational social choice. The malpractice system has three basic goals: (a) reducing rates of iatrogenic injury ("deterrence"), (b) relieving the burden on those who have suffered such injury ("compensation"), and (c) distinguishing blameless from blameworthy conduct ("justice").

In pursuit of these goals, liability is filtered through three functional components of the malpractice system: patient care, legal process, and liability insurance *(8,9)*. Available evidence indicates that all three components fall well short of ideal performance (*see* Table 1). Optimal levels of patient safety are achievable only if the health care system has clear, consistent incentives to gather information about errors, process that information into prevention strategies, coordinate the actions of individual and institutional providers, and communicate effectively with patients. The legal system should provide these incentives by exposing instances of iatrogenic injury, demanding persuasive evidence of avoidability, and awarding damages consistent with loss. The insurance markets should support the legal system by offering peace of mind to careful physicians and making compensation available to victims. Insurers should dispose of meritless claims, help providers improve their safety records, and weed out the worst offenders.

Patient Care

AVOIDABLE INJURIES

The tort reform movement of the 1970s and 1980s was based on two related beliefs: (a) few incidents of actual negligence occur in health care, and (b) most litigation reflects social and financial influences apart from medical quality *(10)*. Subsequent research, much of which is a direct outgrowth of public interest in malpractice reform, largely confirmed the second perception but refuted the first. The Harvard Medical Practice Study (HMPS) reviewed medical records from hospitalizations in New York State during 1984 and looked for associated liability claims; it concluded that roughly six unfounded claims were filed for every meritorious one *(11)*. In a follow-up study, the severity of the plaintiff's condition, not negligence or even medical causation, was the strongest predictor of payment through the legal system for cases evaluated by the HMPS *(12)*. On the other hand, the HMPS reviewers found evidence of negligent injury in 1% of hospitalizations; only one-eighth of these negligent injuries generated lawsuits, and only half of those claims were compensated through litigation. This mismatch between instances of actual negligence and legal proceedings undercuts the deterrent effect of conventional malpractice liability on poor medical care *(13)*.

The HMPS helped alert an innovative group of physicians to serious safety problems in the health care system *(14)*. By the late 1980s, quality researchers had established that medical practice was far less coherent than it had previously appeared and that little data existed linking health care processes to successful outcomes. The patient safety movement grew up alongside these quality improvement efforts, with medical errors demonstrating in salient fashion the need to replace traditional oversight of individual health professionals with a more systematic approach to process re-engineering that matched the growing sophistication of the health care industry. In 1999, the Institute of Medicine (IOM) published its landmark report, *To Err is Human*, and brought patient safety and its cousin, medical quality, onto the national political and policy agenda *(15,16)*.

The relationship between liability reform and the patient safety movement remains unsettled. On its face, *To Err Is Human* envisions a constructive role for institutional liability in promoting system-based safety and criticizes traditional malpractice law primarily for its focus on individual practitioners and, therefore, its chilling effect on efforts to gather and share information about error. However, because the

IOM report confirmed as well as contradicted beliefs held by various constituencies, its implications for liability are often misinterpreted or distorted *(17)*.

For physicians (including some leaders of the patient safety movement), the essence of the report was that safety can best be improved cooperatively by the medical profession through the use of new, self-regulatory methods. The report did not dislodge their belief that malpractice law continued to represent a hostile outside threat. This tunnel vision was worsened by the efforts of some malpractice liability insurers to use "nonpunitive" patient safety theories to bolster old arguments for caps on damages and other traditional tort reforms.

Patients were partly sympathetic to this view because they believed their doctors are well-intentioned, but they also noticed an obvious fact that largely eluded physicians: the IOM report had vindicated longstanding claims by the plaintiffs' bar that the medical profession was ignoring an epidemic of medical error. These discordant reactions may have increased patients' interest in suing and jurors' willingness to find liability *(18)* while blinding the medical profession to liability innovations that could be both affordable and safety-enhancing.

DEFENSIVE MEDICINE

During lulls between malpractice insurance crises, arguments about the pernicious influence of malpractice litigation on overall growth in health care spending (which enjoys a respite much more rarely) have been the mainstay of traditional tort reformers. Certainly, increases in health care costs that do not improve patient safety reduce access to health care at the margin by rendering private health insurance less affordable. However, malpractice insurance premiums and self-funded reserves total only about 1% of annual health expenditures *(19)*. Although this is hardly pocket change in a trillion-dollar health care system, it also does not present a compelling case for reform, especially considering that tort compensation is a transfer payment from provider to patient and not a net social cost.

Therefore, budget arguments for malpractice reform typically extend beyond the direct costs of litigation to "defensive medicine," meaning inducement of health care intended to discourage litigation rather than confer medical benefit *(20)*. Because most filed claims do not reflect underlying negligence and physicians greatly overestimate both litigation and liability risk, there is a good conceptual case for defensive medicine. Many estimates of defensive medicine seem unreliable because they are based on casual extrapolations from physicians' self-reported liability concerns and responses to hypothetical changes in the tort system *(21)*. However, one study examined actual liability exposure and actual health care utilization and concluded that a substantial sum is being spent annually in the United States for defensive reasons *(22)*.

In the present crisis, a different form of defensiveness may have even greater policy significance. There has always been modest evidence that some physicians refrain from performing certain procedures or avoid particular types of patients for fear of being sued, which is called "negative" defensive medicine. However, nothing suggested that this behavior was widespread. This may be changing, perhaps because the monetary costs of liability no longer can be passed through to payers and the public. With malpractice insurers retrenching in many states and applying strict underwriting criteria to potential customers, many physicians are desperate to avoid being sued for fear that it will raise their premiums or jeopardize their coverage.

Some defensive reactions, such as refusing to care for sick children or to perform difficult surgical operations, may be narrowly rational because poor outcomes in those situations indeed correlate with legal exposure. Occasionally, better quality of care may even follow if cases that might be mishandled by generalist physicians in office practice are referred to high-volume specialists (e.g., sending complicated pediatric cases to children's hospitals). In areas with shortages of certain services, however, defensive practice can compromise access to care. Even worse, many efforts at self-protection, such as avoiding poor patients or patients with terminal diseases, have no plausible liability-reducing effect and merely reinforce stereotypes that already burden vulnerable populations *(23)*. Physicians may also expend considerable time and energy trying to predict which patients are more likely to sue, a needless distraction that distorts doctor–patient communication and interferes with the development of a therapeutic bond.

Legal Process

DELAY

The process of resolving malpractice claims is slow. Litigation is a customized enterprise with few economies of scale and strategic incentives for each side to impose costs on the other to pressure settlement. Consequently, administrative expenses consume approx $1.50 for each $1 of actual compensation, which is grossly inefficient compared with first-party health, life, or disability insurance and constitutes a true social cost of the malpractice system *(14)*. On average, more than 3 years elapse between filing a malpractice claim and receiving a final determination. Very large claims typically take longer. Prefiling delays exacerbate the problem, particularly delays for claims involving children, which enjoy liberal statutes of limitations. As a result, some cases remain unresolved for decades. Pennsylvania's patient compensation fund, which began providing secondary coverage for malpractice claims in the 1970s, has yet to formally close the books on a single year of its operations *(24)*.

Delay is implicated in many failings of the malpractice system, perhaps the least important of which is its administrative cost. Patients whose claims are motivated mainly by a desire to understand what happened to them are denied that information for prolonged periods, and patients who were seriously injured by negligence seldom receive compensation when they most need it. Many legitimate smaller claims are not brought or are dropped without resolution because the financial or psychic cost of pursuing them exceeds the potential benefit. As the process crawls along, frustration mounts for both patient-plaintiffs (who want redress) and health professional defendants (who want vindication or at least closure), positions harden, and interactions become increasingly adversarial and unpleasant.

Delay less often places liability insurers and defense counsel at a disadvantage, which is why they allow it, but nonetheless it harms insurance markets. The "long tail" of malpractice insurance—a product of both prefiling and postfiling delay—impairs insurers' ability to accurately estimate their exposure, makes insurer profits dependent on investment yields, and heightens the risk of insurer insolvency prior to claims resolution, all of which increase premium volatility and threaten availability and affordability of coverage during crisis periods.

Finally, delay eliminates any possibility of the liability system supplying effective feedback to the health care system regarding patient safety. A judgment or settlement in a major case 5 or 10 years after an injury occurred is far less capable of conveying useful lessons to the professionals and institutions who were involved in the care being reviewed.

POOR COMPENSATION

The legal system is notoriously poor at compensating injured patients. As noted, most negligent injuries never generate legal claims, whereas payments are sometimes made in cases with poor medical outcomes but little evidence of substandard care. In cases where juries hold defendants liable for actual negligence, damage calculations are often uninformed and unguided, even when judges confront posttrial motions for remittitur. The fact that caps on damages have thus far proved the only way to stabilize malpractice insurance premiums makes matters worse. Statutes may place an absolute cap on total damages (as in Colorado); limit only damages for noneconomic injury such as physical or emotional pain and suffering (as in Ohio); or limit punitive damages (as in North Carolina). As of 2002, 21 states had placed caps ranging from $200,000 to $1 million on noneconomic damages. Noneconomic damage caps have been estimated to reduce the mean payout per claim by up to 40%; the effect on insurance premiums is smaller *(9)*.

Caps have attracted criticism. In particular, flat caps on noneconomic or total damages may be unfair to young or severely injured plaintiffs but fail to constrain overly generous compensation for minor injuries because this compensation remains below the cap *(25)*.

The case of neonatal injury described in the preceding section illustrates three additional limitations of a cap on noneconomic damages as a solution to the current malpractice crisis. First, *economic* damages can still be extremely high when prolonged medical care is required, and the money to pay them has to come from somewhere. Second, calculating those economic damages requires juries to evaluate complex and contentious expert testimony involving medical economics as well as clinical prognosis. Third, pain and suffering awards are increasing partly because long-term survival after serious injury has become more common. The implicit message in limiting damages for future suffering in these cases is that the patient should feel lucky to be alive. This approach is typical of "wrongful birth" claims, where physicians who do not cause but fail to diagnose congenital disease may be liable for the costs of caring for the child but not for its pain or suffering. A similar compromise also may be socially defensible in certain malpractice cases to preserve access to medical care that prolongs life; however, its fairness should be debated openly.

This example highlights the absence of a rational connection between what society invests in health care and what society expects to receive when health care goes awry. In part, this is an inevitable result of funding the costs of malpractice through third-party liability insurance rather than first-party health and disability insurance. Insured health care providers prefer that their carriers pay claims only as a last resort, and patient claimants see no direct link between the generosity of settlements and the cost of health care. The influence of medical cost-containment on the malpractice system is similarly unplanned. Tort reformers cite a 10-fold increase in average annual liability premiums per long-term care bed over the past decade as evidence of a litigation explosion. Rising liability costs for today's skilled nursing facilities are more accurately explained by two health policy developments. First, changes in Medicare reimbursement for acute care hospitals channeled younger but sicker patients requiring real medical treatment into what previously had been merely residential and custodial institutions. Second, public policy decisions at the state and federal level conferred enforceable legal rights on long-term care patients similar to those already in place for hospital patients.

Finally, the adversarial system that governs malpractice disputes often precludes giving plaintiffs satisfaction in forms other than money. In some instances, patients and their families are more interested in having health care providers acknowledge their mistakes and take steps to assure that similar tragedies never happen again *(26–28)*. However, money tends to be the only medium of exchange that malpractice lawyers on either side understand, both for themselves and for their clients. Unlike mediation and other more open-ended approaches to dispute resolution, litigation offers few opportunities for interest-based, as opposed to positional, bargaining *(29,30)*.

Liability Insurance

POOLING AMONG SPECIALTIES

A malpractice crisis is like an earthquake: it strikes unevenly. Even under the most extreme market conditions, only some physicians find liability insurance unavailable or unaffordable. Liability insurance typically is priced according to the frequency and severity of paid claims associated with a physician's specialty and with the community in which he or she practices (i.e., in which a lawsuit would be filed and tried). Therefore, physicians who perform risky surgery on younger patients whose legal damages are potentially great (e.g., orthopedists and neurosurgeons), deliver babies who might suffer lifelong disability (e.g., obstetricians), or diagnose life-threatening but potentially treatable diseases (e.g., mammographers) pay much more for liability coverage than physicians who treat older patients, avoid invasive procedures, or treat self-limiting ailments. These effects are magnified during crisis periods, as carriers abandon marginal markets and customers and apply increasingly conservative assumptions to actuarial predictions for physicians with whom they continue to do business.

Pricing insurance according to legal risk is superficially appealing, but it is illogical on close examination. Like much of the malpractice system, class-rating is a vestige of the historical fragmentation of medical practice, which is reflected in single-line coverage for physicians (hospitals and other corporate providers generally have separate liability carriers or self-insure). From a narrow business perspective, class-rating protects profitability for individual insurers. However, legal risk and social risk are not the same, and regulatory concerns over firm-level solvency can be dealt with in other ways (e.g., guaranty funds).

Modern medicine is a collaborative enterprise; nothing is to be gained by society discouraging physicians from entering high-liability fields such as obstetrics or neurosurgery. In addition, the current system does not offer meaningful incentives for specific physicians to reduce their risk. Experience-rating at the individual physician level is too imprecise to be effective, and the small number of obviously unskilled physicians who should be denied coverage entirely often make use of state-sponsored high-risk pools that were established at a time when repeated malpractice claims were still considered the result of aggressive lawyering rather than bad medicine.

Sharing liability costs to a greater degree among physicians (and other providers) would not threaten private insurance markets through adverse selection. Adverse selection only occurs in voluntary markets, whereas malpractice insurance is either required by state law or by hospitals as a condition of granting privileges. The only plausible justification for class- and geographic-rating is based on fairness, not efficiency: urban specialists often earn more than family practitioners in rural areas. However, this does not explain why some lucrative specialties pay far less for coverage than others and burdens inner city providers more than their wealthier suburban counterparts.

INDUSTRIAL BASE

With most hazardous commercial activities, liability costs are borne in rough proportion to revenue. This lodges responsibility with the wealthiest and, therefore, most efficient risk-bearers, ensures that resources will be available to compensate victims, and reduces hazard levels by building the cost of injury into the price of the product. Medical malpractice law (like tort law in general) links liability to negligent behavior that causes injury. Accordingly, compensation for medical injury is paid mainly by physicians' malpractice insurance because physicians' decisions largely determine what care patients receive and how it is delivered. This made perfect sense when most medical costs consisted of physician time and hospitals were charitable institutions performing a low-technology, supportive role. As medicine has become industrialized—requiring the coordinated application of a range of professional services, technical facilities, and sophisticated products—physician direction has become more difficult and the results of faulty management more costly. Physician services now account for roughly 20% of national health expenditures, creating a trillion-dollar gap between physician revenues and total revenues because of sustained medical inflation. This puts the deterrent objective of liability in tension with the risk-bearing and compensation objectives. Physicians still plausibly control roughly two-thirds of health expenditures through their ordering and referral decisions, but they are insufficiently capitalized to fund insurance costs to an equivalent degree, particularly when the burden falls mainly on a few specialties.

Another byproduct of the preindustrial structure of liability insurance is that focusing on physicians distracts policymakers from an equally important set of concerns affecting hospitals and other medical institutions. Even in crisis periods, primary layers of coverage for institutional providers remain financially viable because they deal with commercial carriers who base premiums on loss experience across a range of revenue-producing clinical activities, they have access to alternative arrangements such as captive insurers and risk-retention groups, and they can self-insure to a considerable degree if necessary *(31)*. On the other hand, institutions in high-exposure states face significant difficulties securing excess coverage, which they keep at high levels to allay shareholder concerns or trustees' fears of personal liability. External shocks to global reinsurance markets, including but not limited to the terrorist attacks of 2001, have significantly reduced available capacity. In this environment, reinsurers are reluctant to devote scarce capital to areas, such as medical malpractice, that are characterized by infrequent but high-dollar losses. This reluctance derives, at least in part, from the publicity that attends occasional jury verdicts against hospitals or HMOs for amounts exceeding $50 million, even if the highest awards are often reduced or the cases are settled for lesser amounts. Recent legislation in New York to repeal periodic payment requirements that were generating extremely high nominal damages and to return to lump-sum awards can be seen as an attempt by hospitals to moderate the tendency of insurance actuaries in a tight market to make worst-case projections.

APPROACHES TO COMPREHENSIVE LIABILITY REFORM

Watching the legislative fight over malpractice reform as portrayed in partisan advertising and the press, one would think that the universe of expert opinion divided cleanly between those who favor $250,000 caps on noneconomic damages and those who oppose them. In fact, the sharpest division is between the stakeholders on one side (both physicians and plaintiff attorneys), who cast the debate in terms of noneconomic damage caps, and the academic community on the other, for whom a damage cap is at best a partial solution to only a subset of critical problems affecting the malpractice system. When the first damage caps were enacted in the 1970s and 1980s, the apparent cause of the malpractice crisis was an epidemic of frivolous claims and excessive jury awards that led commercial liability insurers to withdraw from the market. Research commissioned during that time, including the HMPS, demonstrated a wider range of shortcomings. Considered in light of this improved understanding, caps have the potential to moderate the cost and volatility of liability coverage but may worsen equally troubling aspects of the malpractice system, such as high rates of medical error and inadequate compensation for avoidable injury. Moreover, in today's health care system, caps standing alone may be a less effective long-term response to volatile malpractice coverage than restructuring liability insurance markets (and health insurance markets) to better meet current demands on them. Therefore, most academics believe that some limits on damages are necessary, but only as part of a larger reform effort.

What principles should guide comprehensive malpractice reform? Although many legislative initiatives continue to focus on "first-generation" tort reforms such as damage caps and limits on attorneys' contingent fees, proposals from the academic and policy communities have now entered their third or fourth generation *(32,33)*. One can discern four general approaches around which academic thinking has coalesced. One approach focuses on returning control over malpractice litigation, and ultimately quality assurance, to persons with true medical expertise. The second approach seeks to replace the current fault-based tort system with mechanisms that would simplify the determination of substandard care and causation of injury and facilitate the payment of compensation. The third approach redirects liability risk from individual health professionals to medical institutions, such as hospitals and HMOs, that can bear it more efficiently and effectively. The fourth approach looks to informed consumers to enter into voluntary contractual arrangements with health care providers that modify various aspects of the tort system.

All four approaches have merit. However, the assumptions that underlie each vary, as do their objectives. Some aspects of each remain unresolved, which means that specific proposals that fall within the same approach may be in tension with one another. Finally, some approaches may be based on unstated rationales or have unanticipated consequences.

Expert Resolution

Reforms designed to confer expertise on the malpractice dispute resolution system continue to attract substantial support from physicians, who blame the problems with malpractice litigation on unscrupulous lawyers, naive and impressionable juries, unfocused judges, and deceptive expert witnesses. Proposals to enhance clinical authority in litigation dovetail with theories of patient safety based on voluntary, confidential reporting of medical errors in a "safe," professional environment walled off from the medical malpractice system.

Holding experts accountable to nonexperts is a longstanding problem in society *(34)*, and it is only natural for professionals to resist external review when the public expects it. No form of public accountability is perfect: the legislative process is democratic but erratic; regulatory agencies are expert but bureaucratic, budget-obsessed, and prone to capture; and the civil justice system suffers from a range of familiar infirmities. Market accountability through incentive-based payment systems has greater potential than has generally been appreciated but is incapable of governing all of medicine *(35)*. As a result, modern medicine still enjoys substantial self-regulatory privileges, including aspects of malpractice liability such as a standard of care determined by customary practice. Physicians nonetheless feel that the malpractice system is beyond their control, which compounds the uncertainties they experience from managed care, fraud and abuse oversight, demanding patients, and changing technology.

Two expertise-related reforms that have been widely enacted are certificates of merit and medical screening panels *(36)*. Certificates of merit exist in about one-third of states and require plaintiff attorneys to obtain expert assessments that claims are warranted before filing them. These provisions may be effective in reducing claims filed by inexperienced lawyers, who are less likely than malpractice specialists to weed out meritless cases despite the financial incentive to do so created by contingent fee payment. On the other hand, medical screening panels do not seem to perform well. Panel systems vary in their details, but most involve a hearing before a group consisting at least in part of physicians, with the results of that hearing admissible into evidence should the case proceed to trial. Of the 20 states that enacted screening panel requirements, 11 chose to repeal or invalidate them rather than revise them, often because difficulty finding members created long delays without demonstrably improving the quality of legal claims. Since trials remain rare, and screening panel findings are seldom factually definitive, they also seem to be an inefficient way to improve the quality of evidence at trial in comparison with better use of court-appointed experts, modification of trial presentations, jury learning aids, and the like.

Specialized medical courts have attracted recent attention from physicians and general tort reformers, and bills establishing them have been introduced in Congress and some state legislatures *(37)*. Most proposals contemplate dividing a state into a handful of judicial districts with dedicated, expert trial judges. Proponents argue that these courts would do better than the current decentralized system at managing caseloads, ensuring high-quality evidence, and reaching consistent decisions about liability and damages. On the other hand, specialized courts run risks of becoming politicized, especially in states where judges are elected rather than appointed and in areas where well-financed groups have clearly defined, unvarying interests in a court's outcomes. As Struve observes, one reason the court of appeals for the federal circuit functions well when hearing patent law disputes is that powerful corporations appear as both plaintiffs and defendants. In contrast, in malpractice cases, medical providers and malpractice insurers will always want a specialized court to constrain liability, not expand it. Another caution is that some expertise-based arguments are merely subterfuges for changing the composition of juries. For example, in Pennsylvania the principal effect of the medical courts proposal currently under consideration would be to redistrict the eastern part of the state so that jurors from Philadelphia—who historically favor plaintiffs with respect to both liability and damages—would be mixed with jurors from surrounding counties. Wide variation in jury behavior is an important issue, but it should be addressed openly.

In sum, the malpractice system could benefit from enhanced expertise, but the source of the problem and best reform approach may differ from those commonly cited. Some malpractice claims, especially larger ones, turn on delicate clinical judgments; however, many do not. The mismatch between legal claims and actual negligence has major public policy significance, but claims, findings of liability, and assessments of damages are not random *(25)*. Health care providers are far more likely to be held liable when they provide negligent care than when they provide competent care *(38)*. Detailed facts about medical treatment also reside primarily with defendants. In part because of poor information, most instances of malpractice do not give rise to claims, and many patients go to lawyers because they have not received explanations of their outcomes from health care providers. These considerations argue for educating judges and juries and facilitating their work rather than abandoning them, at least if the goal is to preserve fault-based adjudication of malpractice claims.

Alternatives to Litigation

For decades, proposals have been circulating that would replace malpractice litigation with a faster, cheaper, less adversarial system that could potentially compensate a greater number of injured patients *(39,40)*. Various forms of alternative dispute resolution (ADR) are already in widespread use, although mostly on a voluntary rather than mandatory basis. ADR is intended to eliminate frivolous claims, expedite claims resolution, and reduce litigation expense. Arbitration is a private form of ADR that uses an impartial third party who is usually an expert in the area of controversy. To reduce litigation delay and costs, incentives must exist for the parties in a large percentage of cases to substitute the informal arbitration process for more costly trial procedures. Mediation involves the use of a third party who does not have decision-making authority and does not typically express a direct opinion on the merit of the case but who attempts to facilitate negotiation *(41,42)*. "Early offer" reforms, which penalize plaintiffs if they reject settlement offers that exceed amounts awarded at a subsequent trial, create incentives for timely resolution of claims without involving specific facilitators or forums *(43)*. The Bush Administration supports early offer approaches in combination with caps on damages *(44)*.

Comprehensive reforms that would remove malpractice litigation from the courts entirely also come in various flavors. A pure no-fault approach would compensate for injuries caused by health care regardless of whether conduct by medical providers fell short of optimal. No-fault accident compensation systems for medical injuries exist in New Zealand and Scandinavia but not in the United States. In other proposals, a no-fault approach would be limited to specific types of harm (e.g., obstetrical injuries). Florida and Virginia have adopted no-fault birth injury compensation funds but continue to experience high rates of litigation *(45)*. A neo-no-fault scheme, which can be implemented either by legislation or by private contract, builds on early offer proposals by prohibiting lawsuits against health care providers who acknowledge liability and promptly pay economic damages *(46)*. One might also establish a fault-based state administrative system that would replace the courts in adjudicating medical malpractice claims but retain fault as a basis for liability *(32)*. Finally, accelerated compensation events (ACEs) proposals mix fault and no-fault principles by requiring health care providers to pay prompt compensation upon the occurrence of designated injuries or injury triggers that have been validated by physician experts as typically associated with negligence *(47)*. ACEs are also designed to help health care providers identify areas in which improvement will prevent future injuries and claims.

Most alternatives to litigation include an administrative system for determining damages that does not rely on case-by-case determinations with unfettered discretion. "Scheduling" damages refers to setting amounts or ranges prospectively to make compensation more predictable and fair. Several methods have been suggested. For example, the injured party's noneconomic damages could be fixed based on the severity of injury and the plaintiff's life expectancy *(48)*. Other approaches, which can also be applied within the tort system, include giving juries or other decision makers information on similar past awards or funding service contracts for future necessary care in lieu of cash payments. In addition to optimizing compensation, scheduling damages could reduce administrative expenses by limiting the marginal payoff from additional litigation effort *(9)*.

Comprehensive alternatives to litigation cannot be evaluated in a political vacuum, particularly in terms of budget constraints *(49)*. The key variables are scope (the patients, providers, or injuries subject to the alternative system), exclusivity (whether a choice exists among systems), and generosity (what damages are compensated and at what levels) *(50)*. The most important public policy tradeoff is between affordability and fairness. In the current system, many valid claims are not brought, whereas other claims are overcompensated. The cost to society of compensating more injuries may become unmanageable if the amount of compensation is not limited *(51,52)*. At some point, however, restrictions on eligibility or compensation may become so onerous that the system seems unfair *(25)*. Another critical tradeoff is between administrability and accountability. True no-fault systems (e.g., automobile no-fault) are premised on the notion that the cost of determining responsibility outweighs the benefits, making it more efficient simply to accept accidents as inevitable, compensate victims, and move on.

Understandably, this sits uneasily with the public where medicine is concerned *(53)* because it removes most financial incentives to avoid injuries. For this reason, the more promising proposals from a patient safety (deterrence) perspective (i.e., those that tie compensation to "avoidability" and assess insurance premiums based on experience) are better termed "no-trial" than "no-fault." A third concern is whether one party or the other can appropriate benefits from an alternative system and impose costs on the other party or society by channeling cases into it selectively. For example, plaintiffs may continue to take high-dollar cases to court while using an administrative system only for injuries not worth litigating.

Institutional Liability

As discussed earlier, the assignment of liability for personal injury to corporate entities (e.g., hospitals, pharmaceutical companies) as well as physicians is a byproduct of the industrialization of American health care over the past half-century. Proposals to systematize liability at higher levels of aggregation than individual health professionals (usually referred to as "enterprise liability" or "organizational liability") have become a mainstay of academic thinking about malpractice reform, although they have attracted only occasional support from physicians *(33)*. These range from modest measures encouraging voluntary efforts to coordinate liability among affiliated providers (such as a safe harbor from the federal anti-kickback statute allowing hospitals to provide malpractice insurance to physicians) to sweeping statutory mandates that confer exclusive liability on particular categories of institutional providers.

Institutional malpractice liability has potential advantages over individual liability in terms of patient welfare, loss-spreading, and administrative efficiency. One goal is to get all major health carecontributors on the same page regarding safety. Under current law, (specifically, the Employee Retirement Income Security Act), ERISA shield selectively shelters managed care organizations from liability for personal injury, although courts have evolved serviceable, if not entirely logical, distinctions between benefits determinations and clinical decisions that have resulted in *de facto* health plan liability in many cases *(54)*. Aligning incentives was the premise behind the Clinton Administration's controversial proposal to focus liability on health plans in connection with national health reform *(55)*. The subsequent move away from tightly managed care made the case for exclusive health plan liability less compelling *(56)*. This led to renewed interest in hospital-based enterprise liability *(57)*, particularly as evidence accumulated that most medical errors need to be addressed at the organizational level *(15)*. However, scholars continue to argue that managed care organizations are well-positioned to monitor physician practice *(58)* and promote long-term investment in safety *(59)*. Ideally, health systems would not only integrate their patient safety and risk management efforts but would link these clinical activities to health insurance benefit design and provider payment practices *(60,61)*.

Institutional liability might improve patient compensation by linking the malpractice system to regulatory oversight that promotes early identification of avoidable injury and prompt resolution of potential claims. Because malpractice suits involving severe harm are typically associated with inpatient care and name multiple defendants, consolidated liability can substantially reduce delay and administrative cost when claims arise, particularly if the responsible institution has established a mediation or arbitration system to handle disputes. Large medical institutions may also be better risk-bearers than individually insured physicians because they can diversify legal exposure over the full spectrum of clinical services and have access to a wider array of commercial coverage options and self-insurance vehicles. However, the greater vulnerability of corporate defendants to jury assessments of punitive damages might undercut some of these advantages *(62)*.

The principal barriers to adopting institutional liability are political. The American health care system is still fragmented; therefore, grassroots reforms that benefit large numbers of solo practitioners and small medical groups are most attractive to lawmakers. Further, the lobbying momentum for general business tort reform that typically builds during malpractice insurance crises makes it difficult to incorporate provisions that would expand corporate liability in politically viable legislation. As was clear from the reaction to the Clinton proposal, physicians also worry that institutional liability will further shift clinical authority as well as legal and financial responsibility to corporate organizations. On the other hand, the severity of the current malpractice crisis, coupled with physicians' sense that their autonomy has already been severely compromised, may eventually make the medical profession more supportive of comprehensive institutional liability.

Information and Choice

Information about medical errors and provider responsibility comprises a fourth important category of cutting-edge malpractice reforms.

The economic analysis of medical liability is primarily about information and includes a paradox. Liability rules are necessary only when one party to a contract (i.e., the physician) has better information about the causes and costs of failure than another (i.e., the patient). If patients had perfect information, they would only choose competent physicians with whom they could agree in advance on acceptable criteria for care and for payment. However, in economist Patricia Danzon's words: "Just as imperfect information undermines the efficient functioning of the market, imperfect information undermines the efficient functioning of the liability system ... [and the] fundamental problem [with traditional malpractice reform] is that changing the liability rule does not correct the information asymmetry" (ref. 9: p. 1395). Therefore, an alternative is to focus reform on improving information for both providers and patients and on leveling the playing field between them. Informational measures take two common forms: error disclosure requirements involving specific patients, and publicly available information about malpractice judgments and settlements.

As the Danzon quote suggests, greater transparency regarding medical errors might eventually open private contractual alternatives to tort liability. The primary objection to private contracting has been that patients are poorly informed and are not in a position to weigh the risks when they are in need of medical care. Private contracting would allow parties to contract out of judicially mandated tort rules and might specify the circumstances for liability, the basis for damages, and the rules and forum for dispute resolution (63). Institutional liability can also be structured around private contracts (64), with managed care plans and patients sharing the savings from cost-reducing contractual change through lower premiums for health insurance.

By the end of 2003, eight states had made information about individual physicians' malpractice histories publicly available on the Internet. States vary as to whether they disclose claims, settlements, or judgments and as to whether liability insurers or physicians are primarily responsible for reporting this information to the government. As with physician "report cards," the general principal idea behind Web-based malpractice information is to help consumers make better decisions about their care. Unfortunately, prior malpractice litigation is a poor indicator of physician quality except in extreme cases and can easily be misunderstood by patients. Physicians also may react perversely to the threat of formal reporting because they foresee various unpleasant financial and reputational consequences. For example, the federal law that requires malpractice payments on behalf of physicians to be reported to the National Practitioner Data Bank has been widely evaded, has reduced physicians' willingness to settle claims, and probably should be abolished. On the other hand, a strong argument exists for prohibiting confidential settlements in high-dollar malpractice cases, particularly if confidentiality allows suboptimal safety practices to continue. For example, the potential harm to patients from overworking young physicians in training came to light in the Libby Zion case *(64a)* in large part because the case was brought before a criminal grand jury that issued a public statement, rather than being settled out of view.

In addition to helping consumers make better decisions about care as a private malpractice claim, information can improve system safety by focusing providers on improvement, support the personhood and dignity of victims and families, and foster public debate about the social risks and benefits of medicine *(65)*. For example, trust and other indicators of interpersonal quality are integral to sound medical therapy *(66,67)* and can be jeopardized if health care providers vanish or become uncommunicative of an adverse event occurs. Therefore, information is an important form of compensation and justice for individuals who have been harmed by medical errors. As discussed earlier, the search for explanations motivates many malpractice suits, and assigning blame where blame is warranted may be meaningful to patients and families *(68)*.

There is a trend toward requiring limited disclosure of medical errors and adverse events. The Joint Commission on the Accreditation of Healthcare Organizations somewhat tentatively requires that

"Patients and, when appropriate, their families are informed about the outcomes of care, including unanticipated outcomes" *(Standard RO1.1.2.2).*

A handful of states (e.g., Pennsylvania, Nevada, Florida) have gone farther and mandate error disclosure to patients. In Pennsylvania, comprehensive malpractice reform legislation enacted in 2002 includes a provision stating that

"A medical facility through an appropriate designee shall provide written notification to a patient affected by a serious event..." *(Medical Care Availability and Reduction of Error Act, 40 Pa. Stat. 1303.308 [2002]).*

Using mediation and other structured approaches to communication can help both providers and patients obtain maximum benefit from disclosure mandates (42). The greatest challenge for informational approaches to malpractice reform is the tension between disclosing information and producing information (69). Indeed, the breakthrough insight of the patient safety movement is that creating a "safe environment" in which information can be shared and analyzed is central to improving complex professional processes. Accordingly, patient safety advocates have criticized the malpractice system for chilling information generation and exchange (70,71). Along these lines, it is eminently reasonable to strengthen peer review protections for safety-related information so that true "near misses" and internal analyses are immune from discovery and use in litigation. However, the line between information that should be shared (at least with individual patients) and information that should be reserved for professional quality improvement will never be easy to draw. Therefore, researchers should explore other ways to generate information about medical errors, including public subsidies (72).

PUTTING THE PIECES TOGETHER

Assembling the elements discussed in the previous sections into a coherent malpractice reform proposal has its own set of challenges. Although a detailed analysis of reform vehicles is beyond the scope of this chapter, one can identify three potential sources of change that could overcome political gridlock and more closely link malpractice policy to overall health policy.

Federally Funded State Demonstration Projects

In November 2002, the IOM issued a report entitled *Fostering Rapid Advances in Health Care: Learning From System Demonstrations (73)*, which recommended that the federal government sponsor a series of state-based demonstration projects to test solutions to persistent health policy problems. The report responded to a request from the Secretary of Health and Human Services for innovative approaches to five areas of health care: chronic care, primary care, information technology, health insurance coverage, and liability. The liability recommendation included two options for "patient-centered, safety-focused, non-judicial compensation": provider-based early payment and statewide administrative resolution. Under the first option, provider organizations that elected to participate in a given state would receive limited immunity from tort suits and federal subsidies for excess liability coverage in exchange for establishing systems for detecting and preventing medical errors and promptly paying economic loss and predefined noneconomic damages for identified classes of avoidable injuries. Under the second option, all health care providers in the state would be subject to a federally funded, state-run administrative adjudication system for avoidable injuries based on predetermined schedules of noneconomic damages, which would replace open-ended tort liability.

The IOM recommendation draws heavily on prior research—notably "early offers," ACEs, and enterprise liability—and is sketchy on details. Still, it has five virtues that distinguish it from other reform proposals. First, it explicitly addresses malpractice reform as a component of overall health care reform *(74)*. Second, it recognizes the need for targeted financial support to help relieve the current malpractice crisis. Third, it seeks to make compensation for avoidable injury faster and more predictable and not simply to reduce the volume of litigation. Fourth, it fosters sound medical relationships by emphasizing apology and explanation *(29,75)* and involving patients in the process of identifying and preventing medical errors. Finally, it allows for variation and choice in the health care system rather than assuming that all health care providers, however organized, have the same capacity to improve patient safety *(76)*.

A MALPRACTICE SYSTEM FOR MEDICARE AND MEDICAID

Getting the Medicare program off the sidelines in the malpractice debate is the surest way to connect the liability and health insurance markets and potentially relieve the strain on the health care system created by the current malpractice crisis. The federal Centers for Medicare and Medicaid Services (CMS) undoubtedly recognize the potential for malpractice liability to destabilize access to care for Medicare beneficiaries in the short term and increase program costs in the long term. However, its forays into medical malpractice reform have essentially been limited to supporting the Bush Administration's overall preferences for restrictions on general tort litigation *(44)*.

Instead, CMS should propose a system of error identification, fair compensation, and dispute resolution that would apply specifically to Medicare and Medicaid patients. The framework of such a system could be adopted by administrative rulemaking, although making it fully operational would likely require congressional action. Because of the voting power of the elderly, converting malpractice liability into a Medicare issue is politically perilous. Still, it makes public policy sense. Since its enactment, Medicare has been largely responsible for funding medical progress, promoting industrialization, and (more recently) imposing cost constraints—the forces described earlier as being primarily responsible for the current malpractice crisis: Medicaid has become the largest government health program, and pays for roughly half of

U.S. births. Therefore, Medicare and Medicaid offer the most visible forum for debating the relationship between what America invests in health care and what it expects to receive when health care goes awry. Moreover, a system that provided immediate information and prompt compensation would have substantial advantages over conventional litigation for elderly claimants.

EMPLOYER-SPONSORED HEALTH CARE
AND THE WORKERS COMPENSATION ANALOGY

Employer-sponsored private health insurance covers most Americans. Therefore, the current malpractice crisis affects the ability of businesses to attract and retain workers. Active involvement in health care purchasing also has made business better attuned to employees' experiences as users of medical services. Moreover, industry's continued tolerance of avoidable physical harm in the health care system, especially when it is traceable to faulty systems design, contrasts sharply with general regulatory and self-regulatory changes since the 1960s, which have created a corporate culture exquisitely sensitive to health and safety issues and their relationship to productivity. Finally, health care is an economic engine throughout the country; liability crises reduce present-day prosperity and jeopardize future prospects. To address these issues, the business community could broker a compromise approach to malpractice mirroring workers' compensation, that limits liability but retains incentives for safety and assures prompt, reasonable payment in the event of injury. To accomplish this, employers would need to set aside their parochial interests in using the malpractice crisis as a poster child for general business tort reform to further their workers' interests in safe, reliable health care.

CONCLUSION

This chapter analyzes the first medical malpractice insurance crisis of the 21st century in light of significant changes that have occurred in the health care system since previous crises. It concludes that the established debate over traditional tort reform incompletely defines current problems and leads to ineffective solutions. The chapter began by analogizing the malpractice crisis to the legend of Rip van Winkle and concludes with a different literary parallel. In the 1993 movie *Groundhog Day*, a retelling of Charles Dickens' Christmas classic using a different holiday, actor Bill Murray plays a local weatherman assigned to cover the early February festivities in Punxatawny, Pennsylvania. To his astonishment, he awakens each morning and finds himself reliving the day before, but he is the only person aware that the day's events have already happened many times. Health care providers, payers, and policymakers are experiencing a similar phenomenon in the current reiteration of the medical malpractice crisis and can profit from following the progression of Murray's cinematic character. The first step is to gain insight into the consequences of one's actions and inactions. The second step is to learn that better things happen when one uses those insights to help others rather than to help oneself. Only then does everyday life begin again, and only then does the future look brighter than the past.

ACKNOWLEDGMENTS

The author thanks Columbia law student Daniel Solitro for research assistance and The Pew Charitable Trusts' Project on Medical Liability in Pennsylvania for financial support.

REFERENCES

1. De Ville K. Medical malpractice in twentieth century United States: The interaction of technology, law and culture, Internat J Technol Assessment in Health Care 1998;14(2):197–211.
2. Mohr JC. American medical malpractice litigation in historical perspective. JAMA 2000;283(13):1731–1737.
3. Maurer H. The M.D.'s are off their pedestal. Fortune, Feb.1954:138–186.
4. Silvers JB. The role of the capital markets in restructuring health care. J Health Pol Policy Law 2001;26(5):1019–1030.
5. Viscusi WK. Corporate risk analysis: a reckless act? Stanford Law Rev 2000;52(3): 547–597.
6. Danzon PM, Pauly MV, Kington RS. The effects of malpractice litigation on physicians' fees and incomes. AEA Papers Proc 1990;80(2):122–127.
7. Grumbach K, Peltzman-Rennie D, Luft HS. Charges for Obstetric Liability Insurance and Discontinuation of Obstetric Practice in New York. Report to the Office of Technology Assessment. Washington, DC: Office of Technology Assessment, 1993.
8. Urban Institute. Medical Malpractice: Problems & Reforms—A Policy-Maker's Guide to Issues and Information. Washington, DC: Urban Institute; 1995.
9. Danzon PM. Liability for medical malpractice. In: Handbook of Health Economics, 1B. Amsterdam, The Netherlands: Elsevier;2000.
10. Regan LJ. Medicine and the law. N Engl J Med 1954;250:463.
11. Harvard Medical Practice Study Group. Patients, Doctors, and Lawyers: Medical Injury, Malpractice Litigation, and Patient Compensation in New York. Cambridge, MA: Harvard Univ; 1990.
12. Brennan TA, Sox CM, Burstin HR. Relation between negligent adverse events and the outcomes of medical malpractice litigation. N Engl J Med 1996;335: 1963–1967.
13. Mello MM, Brennan TA. Deterrence of medical errors: theory and evidence for malpractice reform. Texas Law Rev 2002; 80(7):1595–1637.
14. Leape LL. Error in medicine. JAMA 1994;272(23):1851–1857.

15. Institute of Medicine. Kohn LT, Corrigan JM, Donaldson MS, eds. To Err is Human: Building a Safe Health System. Washington, DC: Nat Acad Press, 1999.
16. Institute of Medicine. Crossing the Quality Chasm: A New Health System for the 21st Century. Washington, DC: Nat Acad Press, 2001.
17. Latham, SR. System and responsibility: Three readings of the IOM report on medical error. Am J Law Med 2001;27(2&3):163–179.
18. Brennan TA. The Institute of Medicine report on medical errors—could it do harm? N Engl J Med 2000;342:1123–1125.
19. Rubin RJ, Mendelson DN. Defensive Medicine and Medical Liability Reform: Estimating Costs and Potential Savings. Fairfax, VA: Lewin-VHI, 1993.
20. Bovbjerg RR, Dubay LC, Kenney GM, et al. Defensive medicine and tort reform: new evidence in old bottles. J Health Polit Policy Law 1996;21:267–288.
21. Klingman D, Localio AR, Sugarman J, et al. Measuring defensive medicine using clinical scenario surveys. J Health Polit Policy Law 1996;21:185–217.
22. Kessler D, McClellan M. Do doctors practice defensive medicine? Q J Econ 1996; 111(2):353–390.
23. Burstin HR, Johnson WG, Lipsitz SR, et al. Do the poor sue more? A case-control study of malpractice claims and socioeconomic status. JAMA 1993;270 (14):1697–1701.
24. Hofflander AE, Nye BF, Nettesheim JD. Report on the Medical Malpractice Insurance Delivery System in Pennsylvania. Pennsylvania Trial Lawyers Association, 2001.
25. Mehlman MJ. Resolving the Medical Malpractice Crisis: Fairness Considerations. The Pew Charitable Trusts' Project on Medical Liability in Pennsylvania; 2003 (monograph available at Website: www.medliabilitypa.org; accessed 5/26/04).
26. Beckman HB, Markakis KM, Suchman AL, et al. The doctor–patient relationship and malpractice: lessons from patient depositions. Arch Intern Med 1994;154(12): 1365–1370.
27. Huycke LI, Huycke MM. Characteristics of potential plaintiffs in malpractice litigation. Ann Intern Med 1994;120(9):792–798.
28. Vincent C, Young M, Phillips A. Why do people sue doctors? A study of patients and relatives taking legal action. Lancet 1994;343:1609–1613.
29. Dauer EA, Marcus LJ. Adapting mediation to link resolution of medical malpractice disputes with health care quality improvement. Law Contemp Probl 1997; 60(1):185–218.
30. Fisher R, Eury W. Getting to Yes: Negotiating Agreement Without Giving In. New York, NY: Penguin, 1991.
31. Mello MM, Kelly CN, Studdert DM, et al. Hospital behavior in a tort crisis: observations from Pennsylvania. Health Aff 2003;22(6):225–233.
32. Kinney ED. Malpractice reform in the 1990s: past disappointments, future success? J Health Polit Policy Law 1995;20(1):99–135
33. American College of Physicians. Beyond MICRA: new ideas for liability reform. Ann Intern Med 1995;122(6):466–473.
34. Gold JA. Wiser than the laws?: The legal accountability of the medical profession. Am J Law Med 1981;7(2):145–181.
35. Institute of Medicine. Leadership by Example: Coordinating Government Roles in Improving Health Care Quality. (Corrigan JM, Eden J, Smith BM, eds.), Washington, DC: Nat Acad Press; 2002a.

36. Struve CD. Expertise in Medical Malpractice Litigation: Special Courts, Screening Panels, and Other Options. The Pew Charitable Trusts' Project on Medical Liability in Pennsylvania; 2003 (monograph available at Website: www.medliabilitypa.org; accessed 5/26/04).

37. Howard PK. Yes, It's a Mess—But Here's How to Fix It. Time Magazine, June 9, 2003.

38. Mello MM, Hemenway D. Medical Malpractice As an Epidemiological Problem. Soc Sci Med 2004;59(1):39–46.

39. Sugarman S. Doing away with tort law. California Law Rev 1985;73:555–663.

40. Bovbjerg, RR, Sloan FA. No-fault for medical injury: Theory and evidence. Univ Cincinnati Law Rev 1998;67(1):53–123.

41. Johnson SM. The case for medical malpractice mediation. J Med Law 2000;5: 21–31.

42. Hyman CS, Liebman CB. Using mediation skills to manage disclosure of medical errors and adverse events. Health Aff 2004;23(4).

43. O'Connell J. Offers that can't be refused: Foreclosure of personal injury claims by defendants' prompt tender of claimants' net economic losses. Northwestern Univ Law Rev 1982;77(5):589–632.

44. US Department of Health and Human Services. Confronting the New Health Care Crisis: Improving Health Care Quality and Lowering Costs By Fixing Our Medical Liability System. Online. Available at Website: http://aspe.hhs.gov/daltcp/reports/litrefm.pdf; accessed on Oct. 1, 2002.

45. Sloan FA. The road from medical injury to claims resolution: how no-fault and tort differ. Law Contemp Probl 1997;60(2):35–111.

46. O'Connell, J. Neo-no-fault remedies for medical injuries: coordinated statutory and contractual alternatives. Law Contemp Probl 1986;49(2):125–141.

47. Tancredi L, Bovbjerg R. Rethinking responsibility for patient injury: accelerated-compensation events, a malpractice and quality reform ripe for a test. Law Contemp Problems 1991;54(2):147–177.

48. Bovbjerg RR, Sloan FA, Blumstein JF. Valuing life and limb in tort: scheduling "pain and suffering." Northwestern Univ Law Rev 1989;83(4):908–976.

49. Sage WM. Principles, pragmatism, and medical injury. JAMA 2001;286:226–228.

50. Sloan FA, van Wert SS. Cost and compensation of injury in medical malpractice. Law Contemp Problems 1991;54(1):131–164.

51. Studdert DM, Thomas EJ, Zbar BIW, et al. Can the United States afford a "no-fault" system of compensation for medical injury?" Law Contemp Problems 1997;60(2): 1–34.

52. Studdert DM, Brennan TA. Toward a workable model of "no-fault" compensation for medical injury in the United States. Am J Law Med 2001;27(2&3):225–252.

53. Blendon RJ, DesRoches CM, Brodie M, et al. Views of practicing physicians and the public on medical error. New Engl J Med 2002;347(24):1933–1940.

54. Sage WM. Managed care's Crimea: Medical necessity, therapeutic coverage, and the goals of administrative process in health insurance. Duke Law J 2003; 53: 593–666.

55. Sage WM, Hastings KE, Berenson RA. Enterprise liability for medical malpractice and health care quality improvement. Am J Law Med 1994;20(1&2):1–28.

56. Sage WM. Enterprise liability and the emerging managed health care system. Law Contemp Probl 1997;60(2):159–210

57. Abraham KS, Weiler PC. Enterprise medical liability and the evolution of the American health care system. Harvard Law Rev 1994;108:381–436.
58. Havighurst CC. Vicarious liability: relocating responsibility for the quality of medical care. Am J Law Med 2000;26:7–29.
59. Arlen J, MacLeod WB. Malpractice liability for physicians and managed care organizations. NYU Law Rev 2003;78:1929–2006.
60. Gosfield AG. Making quality happen: in search of legal weightlessness. In: Gosfield AG (ed.), 2002 Health Law Handbook. Deerfield, IL: Clark Boardman Callaghan, 2002.
61. Grol R. Improving the quality of medical care: building bridges among professional pride, payer profit, and patient satisfaction. JAMA 2001;286:2578–2585.
62. Studdert DM, Brennan TA. The problem of punitive damages in lawsuits against managed-care organizations. New Eng J Med 2000;342(4):280–284.
63. Havighurst CC. Health Care Choices: Private Contracts as Instruments of Health Reform Washington, DC: AEI Press, 1995.
64. Sage WM, Jorling JM. A world that won't stand still: enterprise liability by private contract. DePaul Law Rev 1994;43(4):1007–1043.
64a. Asch DA, Parker RM. The Libby Zion case. New Eng J Med 1988;318(12): 771–775.
65. Sage WM. Regulating through information: disclosure laws and American health care. Columbia Law Rev 1999;99:1701–1829.
66. Hall MA, Dugan E., Zheng B, et al. Trust in physicians and medical institutions: what is it, can it be measured, and does it matter? Milbank Q 2001;79:613–633.
67. Hickson GV, Federspiel CF, Pichert JW, et al. Patient complaints and malpractice risk. JAMA 2002;287(22):2951–2957.
68. Rosenthal M, Schlesinger M. Not afraid to blame: the neglected role of blame attribution in medical consumerism and some implications for health policy. Milbank Q 2002;80:41–95.
69. Zivin JG. Pfaff ASP. To err on humans is not benign: incentives for adoption of medical error reporting systems. Columbia University Department of Economics Working Paper, July 2003.
70. Liang BA. The adverse event of unaddressed medical error: identifying and filling the holes in the health-care and legal systems. J Law Med Ethics 2001;29: 346–368.
71. Gostin L. A public health approach to reducing error: medical malpractice as a barrier. JAMA 2000;283:1742,1743.
72. Zivin JG, Pfaff ASP. To err on humans is not benign: incentives for adoption of medical error reporting systems. Working Paper 2002.
73. Institute of Medicine, Fostering Rapid Advances in Health Care: Learning from System Demonstrations, (Corrigan JM, Greiner A, Erickson SM, eds.), Washington, DC: Nat Acad Press; 2002.
74. Bovbjerg RR, Miller RH, Shapiro DW. Paths to reducing medical injury: professional liability and discipline vs. patient safety—and the need for a third way. J Law Med Ethics 2001;29:369–380.
75. Cohen JR. Apology and organizations: exploring an example from medical practice. Fordham Urban Law J 2000;27(5):1447–1482.
76. Studdert DM, Brennan TA. No-fault compensation for medical injuries: the prospect for error prevention. JAMA 2002;286(2):217–223.

INDEX

Dissatisfaction
with medical profession, xii–xiii
Dissecting aortic aneurysm, 94
Distractions, 66–67, 67
Doctors. *See* Physician(s)
Doctors Company (TDC)
breast cancer claims, 154–163
pap smear litigation, 167–179
Doctrine of autonomy, 141
Doctrine of vicarious liability, 90–91
Documentation, 97
anesthesiology, 120–121
emergency medicine, 103–104
nursing notes, 104–105
patient explanations, 38
plastic and reconstructive surgery medical liability,
185–186
template charts, 104
Double-dipping, 237–238
Double-negatives, 56
Dress
physician witness, 47, 60
Drug addicts
emergency room, 112
Ductal carcinoma *in situ* (DCIS)
low-grade, 161–162
misdiagnosis, 162
Duty, 16–17

E

Early offers, 273
program, 240, 241
reforms, 266–268
Economic damages, 259
Economic loss, 16
Economy
downturn in, 234
Edema of preeclampsia, 149–150
Electronic fetal heart rate monitoring, 144
E-mail, 87
patient–physician communication, 80–81
E-medicine
physician's office, 75–87

Emergency Medical Treatment and
Active Labor Act
(EMTALA), 106–107
Emergency medicine, 101–113
communication, 102–103
documentation, 103–104
lack of English, 103
Emergency subject matter
online communications, 84
Emotion-laden words, 67
Employee Retirement Income Security Act (ERISA), 204, 268
Employer-sponsored health care
workers compensation analogy,
274
EMTALA, 106–107
Endotracheal intubation
emergency room, 111–112
End-tidal carbon dioxide monitors,
116
English
lack of
emergency medicine, 103
Enhance expertise, 265
Enoxaparin (Lovenox)
epidural hematomas with, 130
Enterprise liability, 241, 268, 273
hospital-based, 269
Epidural abscess
emergency room, 111
Epidural blocks, 130
Epidural hematoma
after epidural block, 129–130
ERISA, 204, 268
ERisk guidelines, 82–85
fee-based online consultation,
85–86
ERisk Working Group, 82
Errors
diagnostic
breast biopsy malpractice
claims, 162
disclosure mandates
Pennsylvania, 271
interpretation

No-fault accident compensation
systems, 266–267
No-fault birth injury compensation
funds, 266–267
No-fault label, 240
Noneconomic damages, 16
caps on, 216, 237
flat caps on, 259
recoverable
limitations on, 18–19
Nonmeritorious litigation, 206, 210
Nonpunitive patient safety theories,
256
Nonverbal expression, 68–69
Nuisance settlements, 211
Nurse–physician communication
problems of
cases of, 70–71
Nursing notes
documentation, 104–105

O

Obstetrics
anesthesia disasters, 127–128
hemorrhage, 147
malpractice, 139–150
Obstructive sleep apnea, 134–135
Occupational Safety and Health
Administration, 90
Office anesthesia
anesthesia disasters, 128–129
Ohio
MICRA-like reforms, 214
On-call physicians, 79
Online communications eRisk
Guidelines, 83–85
Online diagnosis and treatment
vs fee-based online consultation
eRisk guidelines, 86
Operating expenses
for insurance company, 4
Operating room fires, 131–132
Oral deposition, 29–30
Oregon
tort reforms, 215

Organizational liability, 268
Oropharyngeal airway fires, 132
Outlier verdicts
cost amplification of, 205
Oxytocin
for obstetric hemorrhage, 146

P

Pain
management, 95
narcotic postoperative medication, 134–135
Pal plaintiff attorneys, 58
Pap smears
access to threatened, 220
alerting physicians about inherent false-negative rate, 174
court issues, 175–176
failure to detect abnormal cells, 172
failure to recognize unsatisfactory, 172–173
false-negative, 168
hyperchromatic crowded groups
of cells, 172
importance, 170–171
interpretation errors, 173–174
liability, 174–175
limiting, 170–171
managed care, 170
litigation, 167–179, 169t
long-term solutions, 177
preventative measures, 176
sources of error, 171–173
Partial summary adjudication, 30–
31
Patient approach, 37–38
Patient care, 255–257
Patient confidence and trust, 234
Patient dignity, 92
Patient expectations
Internet-based care, 80–81
plastic and reconstructive surgery medical liability, 188
Patient explanations
documentation, 38

About the Editor

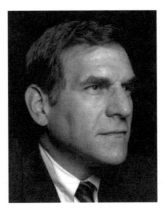

Dr. Anderson is a medical oncologist who practiced for more than 20 years at Scripps Hospital in San Diego where he was also a clinical professor of medicine at the University of California San Diego. He is currently chairman and chief executive officer of The Doctors Company, a national physician-owned medical malpractice insurance company.